Author

Jennifer Young has a BSc (Hons) in biology and is an associate member of the Royal Society of Medicine. She is a qualified nutritional therapist, and an experienced microbiologist, aromatherapist, beauty therapist and product formulator.

With two postgraduate qualifications in health-related fields, she has been accepted by the courts as an expert witness for occupational health cases and has been active in medical research.

Jennifer works with cancer patients to help them to recognise themselves as they go through treatment. Her main interests are skincare and beauty. She is the creator of the Defiant Beauty collections and founder of www.beautydespitecancer.co.uk.

First published in 2015 by

Lotus Publishing

Apple Tree Cottage, Inlands Road, Nutbourne, Chichester, PO18 8RJ

Cover Design and Text Layout

Martin Young

&

Kenteba Kreations (www.kentebakreations.com)

Model Photography Claudio Sardonne

Photography Keating Mary

Stock Images www.shutterstock.com

Printed and Bound in the UK by Bell and Bain Limited

British Library Cataloguing-in-Publication Data

A CIP record for this book is available from the British Library

ISBN 978 1 905367 59 7

JENNIFER YOUNG

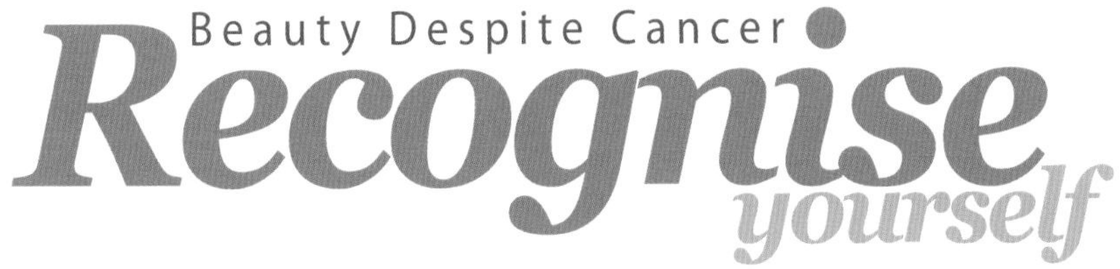

Contents

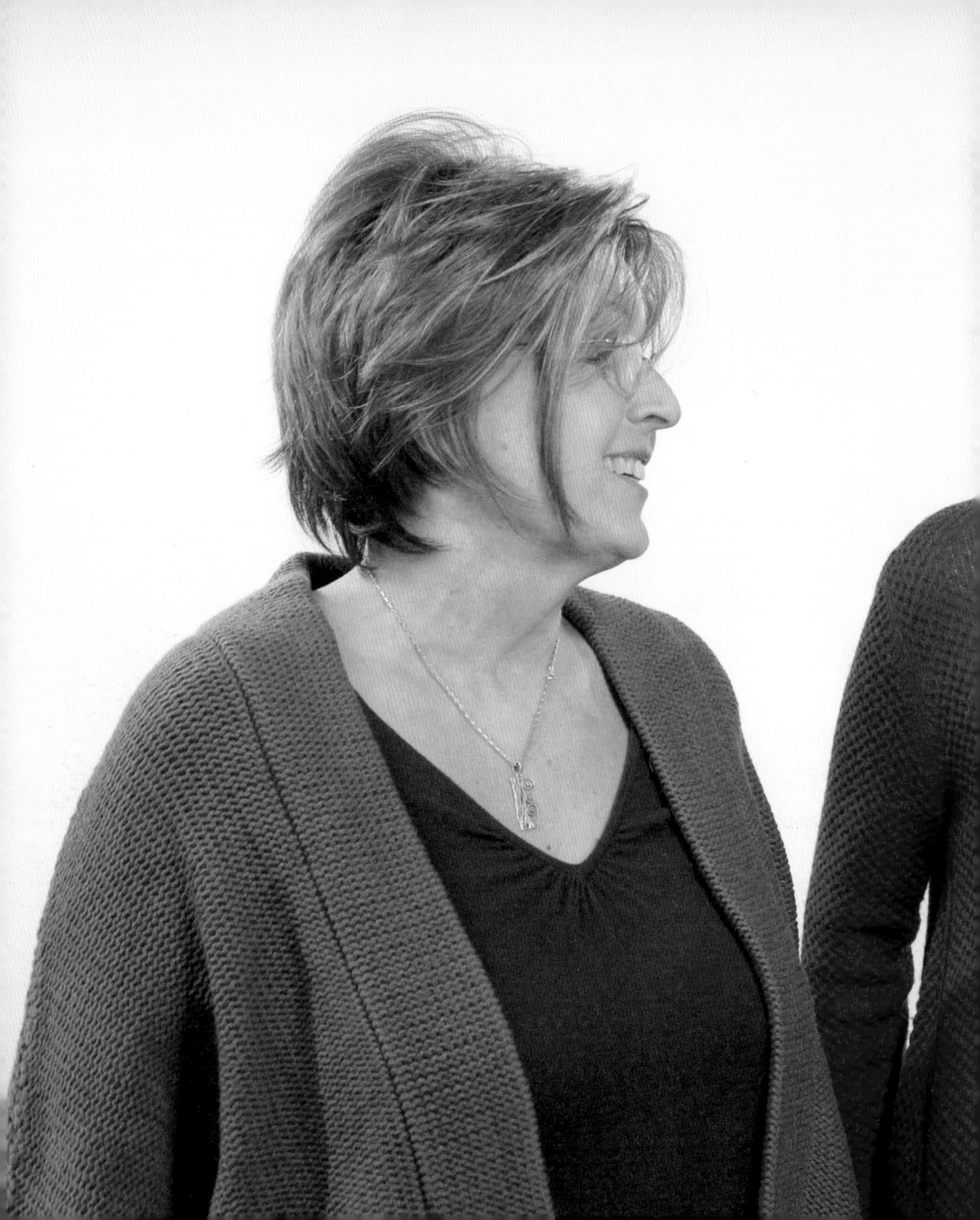

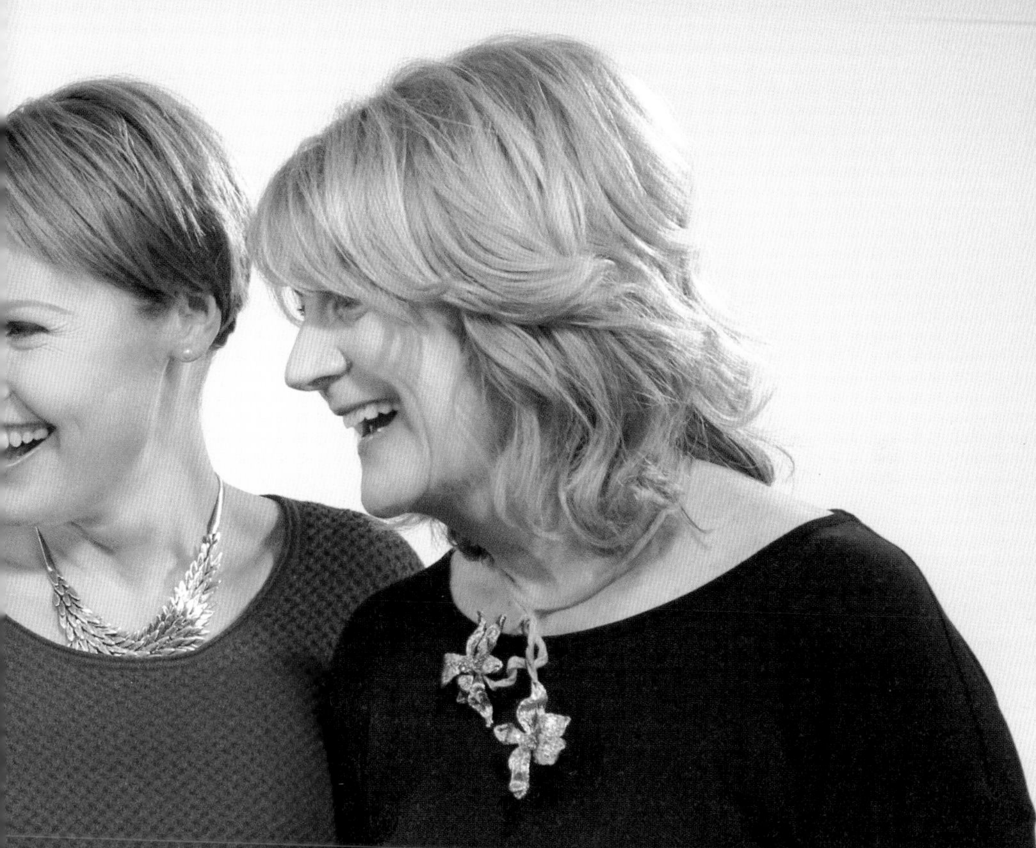

Preface

Preface

'Women don't stop being women when they are diagnosed with cancer.'

I often find myself saying this as a way of explaining why I founded www.beautydespitecancer.co.uk and why I created the Defiant Beauty skincare and beauty collections for cancer patients. It is also the reason I have written this book.

You didn't stop being a woman when you were diagnosed with cancer but you might have stopped feeling like one and being treated like one.

The purpose of this book is to help you to put aside the concerns that you have about your changing appearance. If you are worried about how best to dress your new body shape, read on; ditto if you want to know how to choose the skincare for your changed skin. Are you looking for ideas on how to enhance your eyebrows or eyelashes? Learn how to get the most from your make-up, what to look for in a wig and how to look after it.

It’s not all about how you look – we have some great advice from health professionals about how to recognise yourself and deal with all that you are going through.

The team at Beauty Despite Cancer is unique. Our writers have experience and expertise – here, both are shared with you.

Jennifer Young

www.beautydespitecancer.co.uk

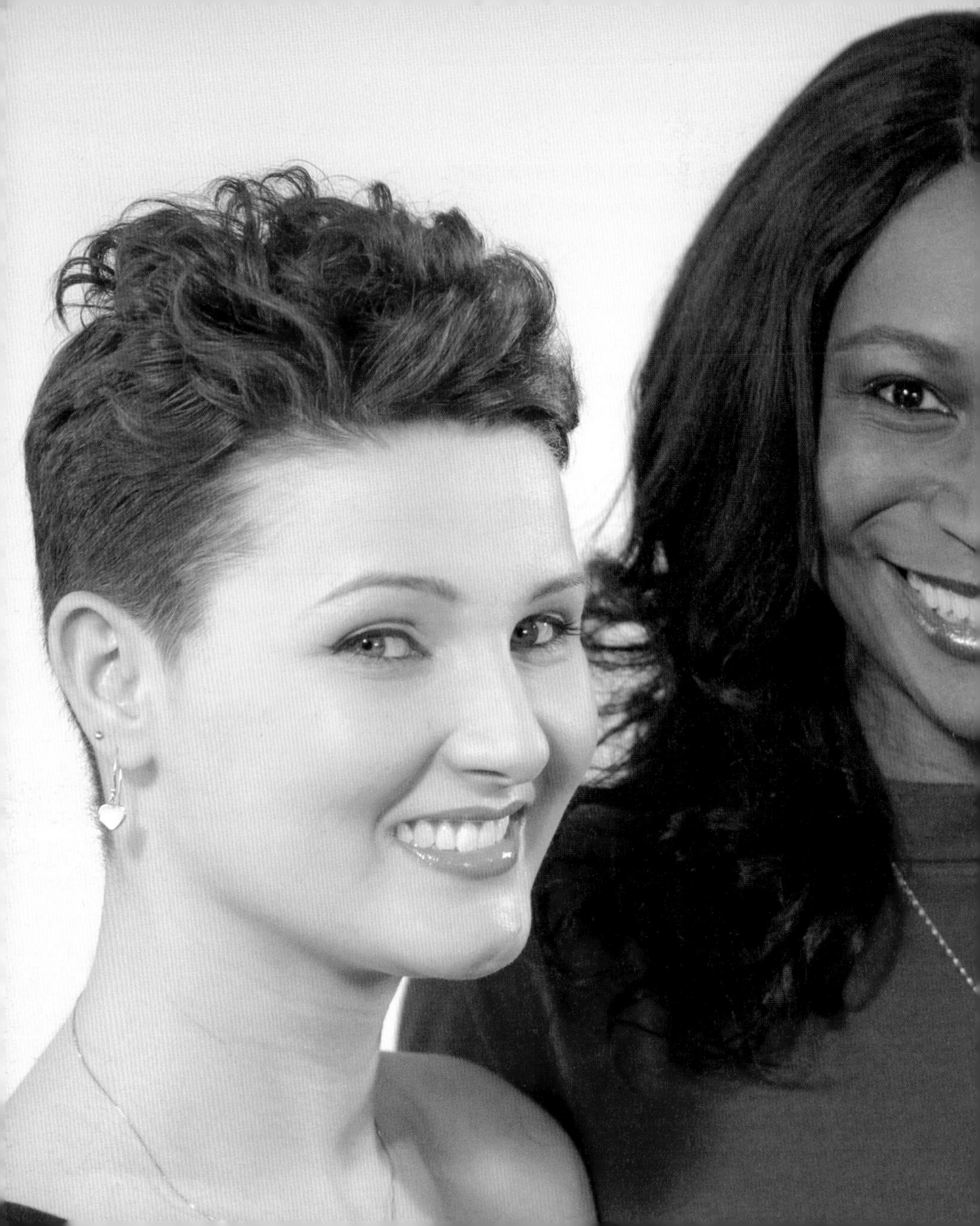

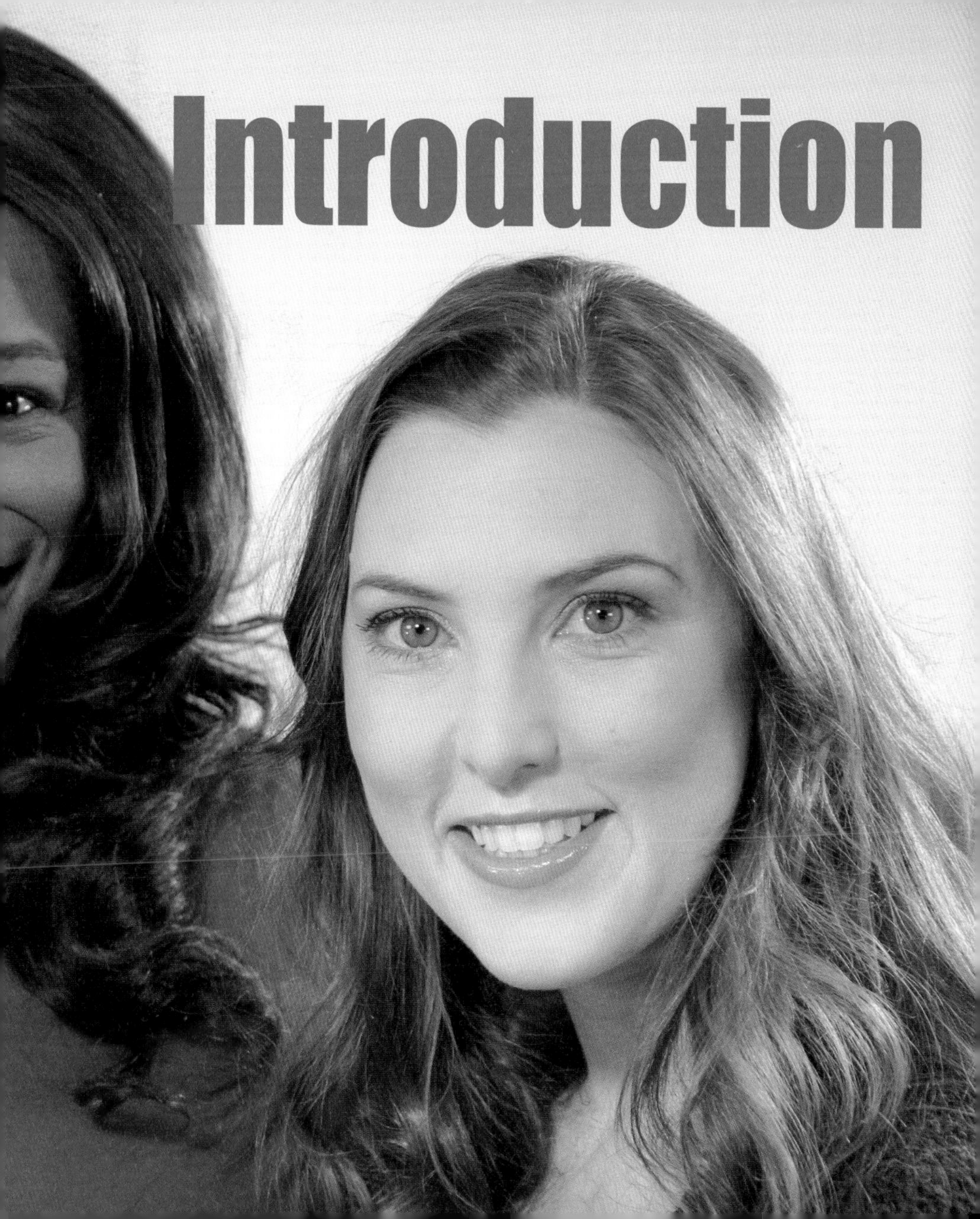

Introduction

Introduction

'Do you have anything for cancer patients?'

This is the question that started it all. Some ladies asked me 'the' question at my local cancer centre. They were opening a beauty and wig salon on the chemotherapy ward and they wanted a skincare range that met their needs. I was asked to help.

The ladies going through treatment and some who had recently finished treatment, along with the lead nurses for chemotherapy and radiology, formed a team; we all worked together, within the guidelines that they had developed, to create a skincare collection that was luxurious and effective. Defiant Beauty was born, at our local NHS hospital.

I thought that my involvement was over when the products were delivered. I had no intention of offering my new skincare collection from anywhere other than the salon on the ward.

It seems that my plans were misguided, as my determination to help women to recognise themselves has evolved way beyond our skincare and beauty products.

It was clear that many of those going through treatment wanted help with appearance-related issues. There was no one to help. The website Beauty Despite Cancer fills that gap, thanks to our wonderful team.

Hopefully, this book goes even further and tells you all you need to know.

I am now proud to be able to answer: 'Yes, we have lots of things for cancer patients.'

Photographs

As if writing a book weren't enough, I was challenged to use 'real people' for the images that are used throughout it.

Many of the visitors to www.beautydespitecancer.co.uk felt that this book would not be 'authentic' unless those pictured on the cover had been through or were going through treatment. I had no idea how I could achieve the goal that I had been set. Typically, I decided to give it a go.

Within weeks I had 15 models, a very highly regarded photographer, make-up artists and hair stylists who are used to working with A-list faces, and a well-known clothing brand on the team. All volunteered their time without charge. I can't thank them enough.

I didn't know how I would get a cover shot but, thanks to the kindness of others, I have more than enough images to fill the book. All of the models you see in this book had been through or were going through treatment at the time of the shoot.

You can read more about the photo shoot in Appendix 1.

Facing the World

You are reading this book. You are looking for help to maintain your appearance as you go through treatment. You probably don't need me to tell you that you are concerned about everyone knowing your medical history as soon as they see you and that you are worried about losing your hair.

You might, however, need me to tell you that you aren't the only one. I have spoken to so many women who believe that they, alone, are thinking about their appearance. Like the others, you probably feel that you should be concerned about 'far more important' matters.

Let me reassure you:

You are not the only one.

The medical team have your back regarding the other 'important' matters.

You are in control of your appearance.

Shall we get started? There is so much to cover.

Men

A Quick Word for Men

Guys – it's OK for you to read this book too. Many men going through treatment feel reluctant to ask for help with appearance-related matters. It's OK to be concerned about a changed appearance and it's OK to seek information to help. I am often asked if I have products for men, and many of the visitors to our website are men.

Most of the information in this book applies to men too and some of it is included specifically for you. Alternatively, you might be reading this because you are living with someone going through treatment and you want to understand and to help. In both cases, I hope that you will find this book useful.

HAIR

'I just sort of sat there absolutely stunned, to think that I had to have chemo and initially, and I will be honest with you, my first thought was, "oh my God I'm going to lose my hair," I didn't think about being sick, I didn't think about anything else, "my God I'm going to lose my hair.[1]"'

Hair

Hair loss is often rated as one of the most common, feared and traumatic aspects of chemotherapy.[1]

'Will I lose my hair?' is one of the first questions asked of oncologists after being diagnosed.[2]

Fiona Macrae was diagnosed when her son was just a few months old. Her first thought? *'Oh my God, I'm going to lose my hair'*; concerns about her son came seconds later.

The Good News

- You will be told if you are likely to lose your hair.
- Your hospital might be able to help you keep your hair, or at least some of it.
- There are many ways in which you can prepare for hair loss.
- You can disguise your hair loss far more effectively than you think.
- Not all chemotherapy results in hair loss.[2]
- Your hair will grow back.

You know you are going to lose your hair – what should you do? There is no right answer to this question. Jo Taylor has twice lost her hair to chemotherapy:

'It was traumatic when I lost my hair the first time. It came out in clumps in the shower. I sobbed for days. This time, losing my hair hasn't been any easier but I have taken it more into my own hands – firstly having it cut short. Everyone told me it suited me short when it grew back last time.

'It was easier for us all when I had it cut short before chemo. The change wasn't as drastic as last time and I was in control. I went from my hair, to long hair, to shaved hair on my own terms.'

Many women decide to take control back into their own hands[1] and have their heads shaved when they start to lose their hair, at the point of diagnosis or soon after.

The nursing team at Clatterbridge Cancer Centre have some great practical suggestions. They advise patients to invest in a hairnet when chemotherapy starts. The nets were described to me as the kind that showjumpers wear. I would have described them as 'the nets my aunties used to keep their perms in, back in the day'.

The net catches any hair that falls. The Clatterbridge team recommend that patients use the net overnight, and throw it away without looking at it, thus avoiding the trauma of seeing their lost hair.

Celebrity stylist Maximiliano Centini works with clients as they go through treatment. Max finds that he acts as an adviser as well as a stylist:

'Reassuring the client is the first priority. Following that, we establish clear steps or goals regarding the hair's recovery. No matter how much I tell a client not to worry, or that she is beautiful, she will be extremely upset when the hair begins to fall out.

'It is important to develop a step-by-step plan of how to manage not only the hair loss but also the regrowth. I remind the client that her hair will grow back and discuss the styles I believe would suit her. We play with the ideas, get her involved and keep her focused on the

next stage. This gives us something to work towards. We celebrate each milestone with something special like a free treatment and work together towards the next phase.'

You may be concerned about how your hair loss will impact your children or grandchildren. Appendix 2 contains some advice from Lyndsay Dobson, a specialist family therapist.

Men

Guys – please don't feel as though you cannot mourn the passing of your hair. Please don't feel that you cannot seek out a wig, look after your scalp or access any of the services that you might think are there for women.

In these pages I have written about hair loss and given it a very female focus – this section, gentlemen, is for you. It's OK to want your hair and to take steps to camouflage your hair loss.

The research that I have discussed in the previous pages, as is often the case, tells us all what we already know to be true. The following statistics are a surprise to me. They have made me realise just how much we exclude men when considering changed appearance.

Help is available for you, gentlemen. Sadly, and unjustifiably, you might have to work a little bit harder to find that help than your female counterparts.

If you feel more comfortable with the idea of having a tattoo than wearing a wig take a look at 'Cosmetic Tattooing' in Chapter 2.

Semi-permanent eyebrows are created using a process similar to tattooing (the ink is not as deep as it would be for a longer-lasting tattoo). The same technique can be used to create 'stubble' and an illusion of shaved hair on the head. More and more semi-permanent make-up artists are offering this service.

Follow the advice given in Appendix 4 when choosing your therapist and make sure you discuss your plans with your medical team. It is unlikely that they will agree to this being done once treatment has commenced. A reputable therapist should refuse to work with you when you are actively in treatment. This is discussed further in Chapter 2.

MALE HAIR LOSS

Of those suffering from hair loss

60% would rather have more hair than **money and friends**

47% would spend their **life savings** to regain a full head of hair

30% would **give up sex** if it meant they would get their hair back

Source: http://www.statisticbrain.com/hair-loss-statistics/

Cooling

Cooling

'Cooling' can help to prevent and reduce some of the appearance-related side effects of chemotherapy. There are special caps designed to reduce the flow of blood to the hair follicles.

Chemotherapy drugs are transported by the blood. Therefore a reduced blood flow to the scalp means less chemotherapy exposure for the hair follicles, which, in turn, can lead to less significant hair loss.[3–5]

Cooling is not appropriate in all circumstances, and you will need the consent and support of your medical team in order to use cooling caps, gloves and slippers. Cooling gloves and slippers are covered in detail in Chapter 3.

Prof. Robert Thomas tells us that the conditions for which cooling is not appropriate are:

- Cutaneous lymphoma
- Cutaneous leukaemia
- Brain metastases
- Skull bone metastases.[2]

Please remember that Prof. Thomas isn't familiar with your particular condition and that your medical team are. They may decide that cooling isn't for you, even if you don't have the conditions listed above.

That aside, if you are able to use cooling equipment, the research has shown that you are more likely to retain your hair if you use a cooling cap.[3–5]

For a variety of reasons, many hospitals do not offer cooling: some because patients don't like the experience, others because cooling means that patients are on the ward for longer. Cooling is an extra job for nurses and care staff; many hospitals simply do not have the resources to support all patients through cooling. Moreover, cooling equipment is expensive and many hospitals do not have a sufficient budget to allow them to offer the service.

There are two types of cooling cap – one attached to a small air-conditioning-type unit, and the other resembling a head-shaped ice pack. If the ice-pack type is used at your hospital, typically three caps will be used per session.

'At Elstree Cancer Centre, all patients for whom it is medically appropriate are offered a cooling cap. They are given meds before it is fitted, to help them to sleep through chemo, their chair is reclined and they are tucked in with a duvet.'

Alina, Breast Cancer Care nurse

Cooling is not a cheap option for your hospital. Please be understanding if they are unable to offer it, or if they are only able to offer cooling to certain patients. Many private hospitals offer cooling to all for whom it is not contraindicated. They may also offer additional services that make cooling more bearable.

If you have a choice of treatment centres and cooling is important to you, discuss it with your medical team.

Everyone seems to feel differently about their experience of cooling. Remember Fiona, who was diagnosed when her son was a few months old? She was able to use a cooling cap and kept most of her hair. Fiona describes the cooling cap as *'not the most pleasant experience'*, but she continued to use it as she desperately wanted to keep her hair. She didn't want to be the '*cancer patient pushing a pram*':

'I didn't want to face that sympathy from strangers and I didn't want to have those conversations. I wanted to be able to take my baby for a walk and have baby-centred chats like all other new mums.'

Our great friend Ismena Clout pulled no punches when describing her experience of cooling caps. She tried them only once and not for an entire session. Ismena, who faced her prolonged and repeated cancer treatments with bravery, determination and humour, decided not to endure the 'head freeze' that accompanied the caps.

Please bear in mind that cooling might not be an option for you, either because it is inappropriate for your condition or because your hospital doesn't offer it.

'Day one of chemo – trying the cold cap made for a welcome distraction. The nervous sighing turned to total hilarity – I looked like a jockey about to race in the Derby. I couldn't hear anything, which proved even more amusing, since my mother (who seems to have been going deaf in old age for the last ten years) and I made a proper pair, yelling at each other across a room the size of a postage stamp! I had that familiar childhood sensation of slurping a McDonald's milk shake too quickly – "brain freeze". My head throbbed for a good few hours! Needless to say, that was my one and only experience of a cold cap.'

Sam Reynolds, Surrey

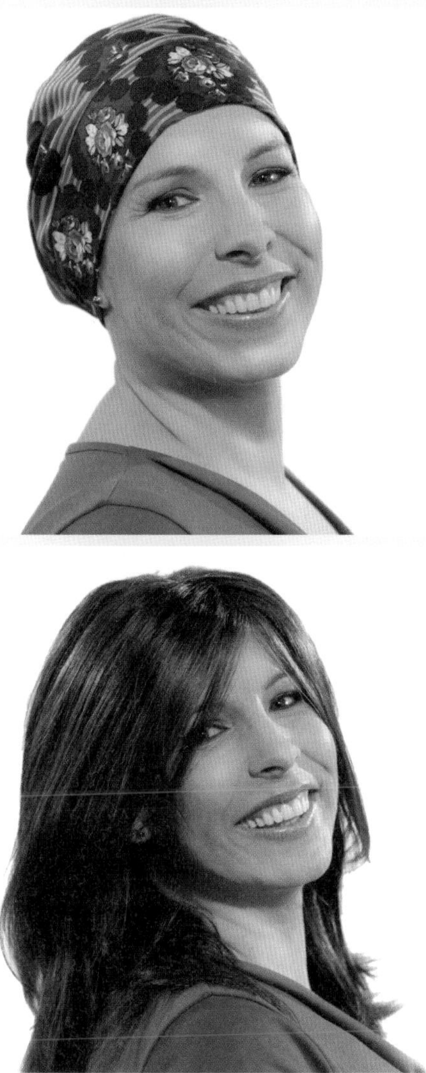

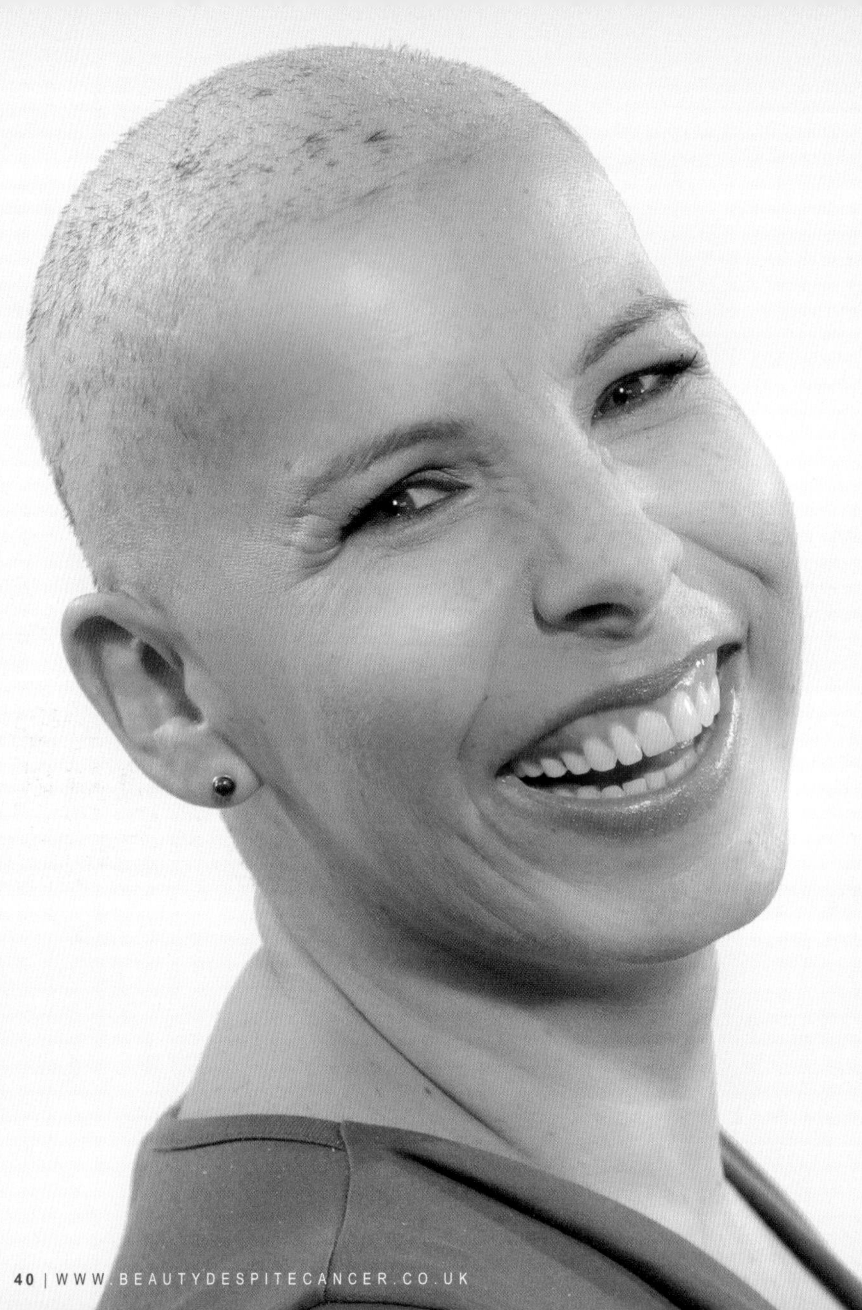

Scalp

Scalp Care

Before we look at head coverings, a few words about your scalp. You've not had to look after your scalp in a long while. You've not seen it in ages. Scalp care is not something you have practised in the past, but it is a skill you should acquire.

Many scalps are prone to breakouts and can become itchy, sore and tight. It gets hot under head coverings.

You can avoid these conditions by following our scalp care routine. Take some advice from Julie Sangster of the Riah Group and treat your scalp as an extension of your face. Don't neglect it.

Typically, scalps can become hot, tight and sore. Caring for your scalp will improve its condition. If you need to cool down when you are out and about, find somewhere private to use a cooling spritz.

Scalp Care Routine

Cleanse

Use a natural cleansing balm to clean your scalp. It is undercover most of the time and bacteria can grow in the humid conditions between you and your wig.

'I always carry soothing oil with me. If my scalp feels tight or itchy I nip to the loo, whip my wig off and apply some oil. The relief is instant.'

Debbie, Aberdeen

Gently exfoliate

Use a hot cotton cloth or an exfolitaing sponge to remove the balm. Dry skin cells will be removed along with the balm. Exfolitaing your scalp can reduce itchiness.

Tone

Have a quick spritz at hand to cool the area and then leave to dry.

Moisturise

If your scalp has been getting tight, apply a small amount of soothing oil and allow it to be absorbed before replacing your wig.

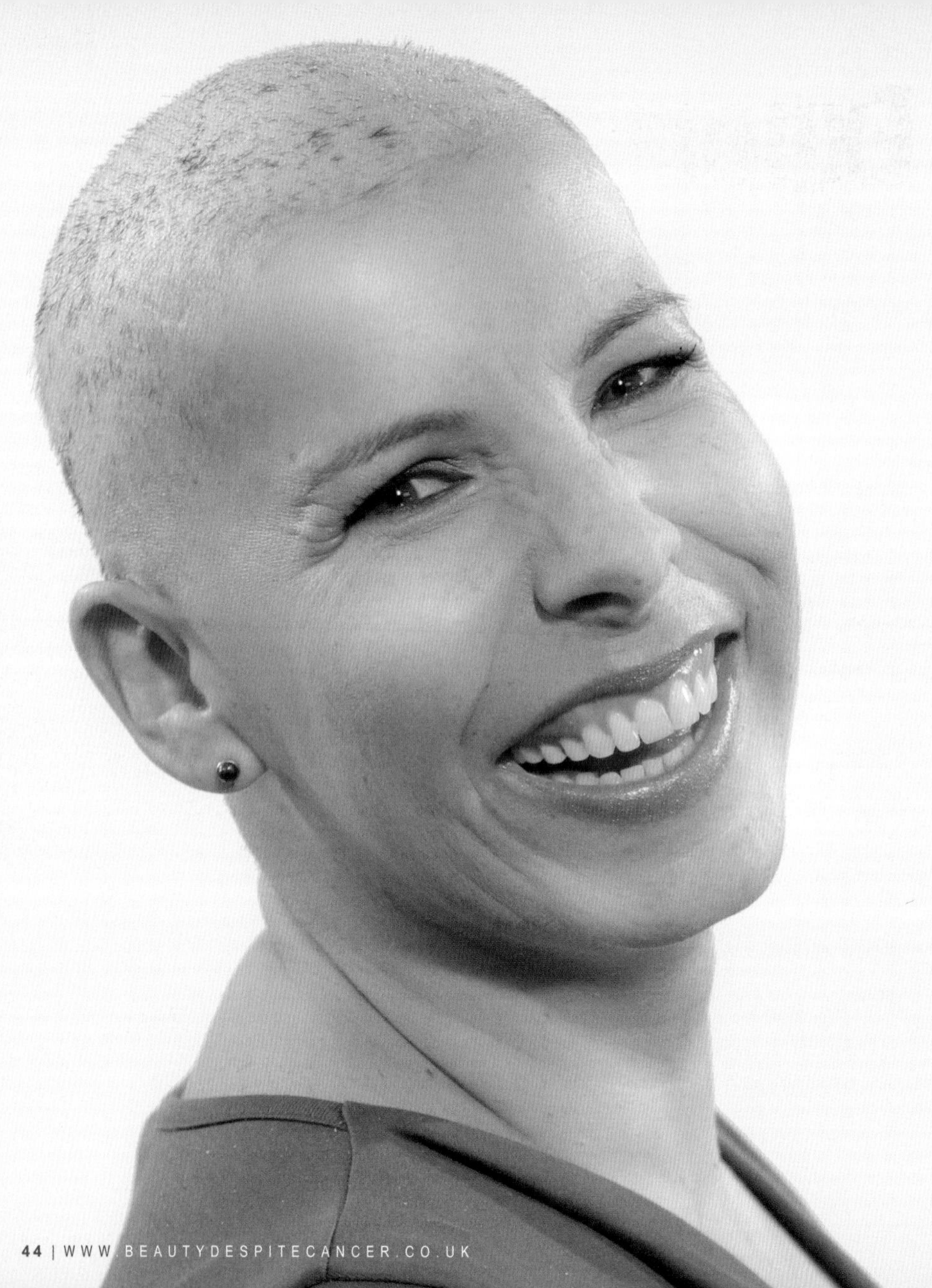

Expert advice

Cleanse, tone and moisturise

Use a cooling spritz if your scalp gets too hot

Refreshing your wig between washes could help to prevent breakouts

Use a soothing oil if your scalp remains dry after your scalp care routine

Give your scalp 'time off' from your wig

Carry an oil or a spritz with you so that you can cool and soothe when you are out and about

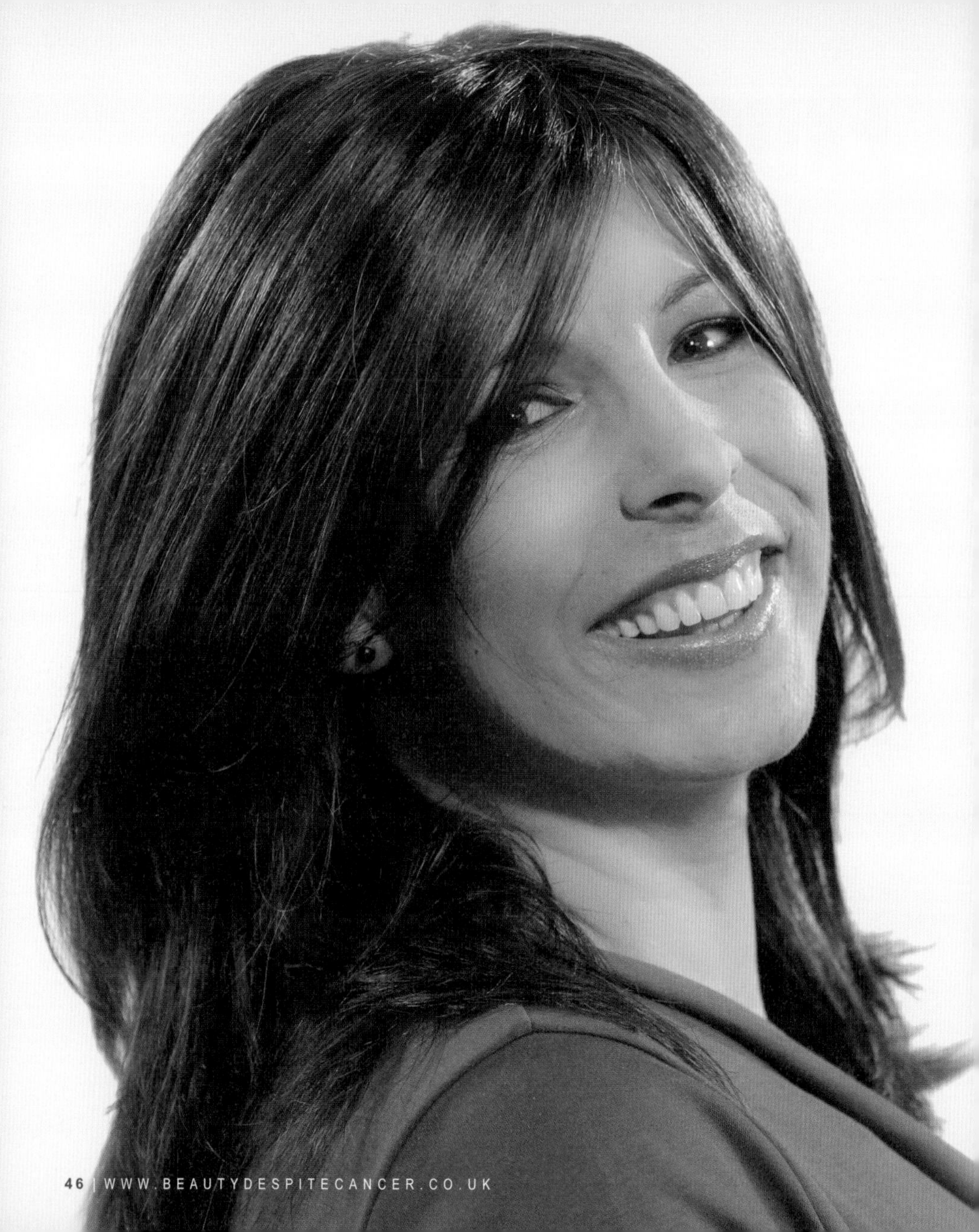

Wigs

Wigs

Audrey Ball of London's Esteem Consultancy, who was the wig stylist for our photo shoot, has extensive experience of wigs. She has had alopecia for 30 years and offers the following advice on choosing your wig (also known as a 'hair system'):

'The right wig for you is the one that makes you feel like yourself again. There is more to it than the look. It has to be physically right. You should look for one that is the right colour, style and quality. Consider the movement of the hair and, more importantly, how it makes you feel when you see your reflection.

'There is no right, only what is right for you.'

Don't feel that you have to choose a wig that is like your hair. Audrey advises that, as you are wearing a wig on medical grounds, you should opt for a good-quality wig that is close to your natural hair colour and you should experiment with style.

When to Have Your Wig Fitted

All of the experts say the same thing: have your wig fitted as soon as you are diagnosed.

Anne Roche of Roches, Dublin, became a wig fitter after recovering from her treatment for cancer. Her dad started the family business after his wife (Anne's mum) lost her hair as a result of treatment for ovarian cancer. Anne asks all her clients to come to see her before they start treatment:

'An early visit takes some of the fear away and reassures women that they can wear a wig without looking as though they are wearing a wig. The wig may need resizing after hair is lost so that it isn't loose. This is part of the service offered by good wig fitters.'

It is an expert's job to make sure that a wig is fitted correctly. Visit a wig fitter and hand over responsibility.

There are two basic rules for correct fit:

1. The hairline should be four fingers above the eyebrow, or thereabouts.

2. The temples of the system should fit comfortably over the ears.

Getting the hairline right is the most important thing for you to do when you are putting your wig on. The four-finger rule will help.

Anne has some tips for wig wearing:

- After brushing your wig with the correct brush, use your fingers like a comb (in the general direction of the wig), to break up the hair and make it look more natural.
- Add some extra movement and interest with wax or gloss. This will create texture and definition, but do not use anything sticky, as you need to avoid a build-up of product in your wig.
- Putting a few layers in your wig can create some natural movement.
- If you feel that your wig has too much hair, it can be thinned out or you can get a finer wig. You can change the colour and style of your hair, but if you go from

fine hair to a wig with thick hair, people will know it isn't your own hair.

- Highlighted wigs tend to look more natural, as the hair looks less dense.
- Wigs that have roots coming through look incredibly natural, just like when you are due a colour, rather than always looking like you have just walked out of the hairdressers.
- Accessorise your wig with scarves or hair jewellery. It changes the look of your wig and definitely fools people. When clients come to the salon with scarves on their wigs, I really have to wonder if it is their wig or their own hair growing back.
- If your wig has any length, create a messy up-style using a grip to hold up your hair. I say 'messy' because you need to leave a fine line of wig hair down on your neck and hairline to camouflage the wig hairline. If your wig is fibre, up-styling will also give it a break from the

friction frizz that happens when fibre hair rubs against your clothes.

- You can make your wig look finer by putting it behind your ears, but leaving a tiny lock in front of your ears to cover where your locks would be.

My favourite wig was being worn at one of our hospital-based pamper sessions: it was black with a purple stripe. The lady wearing it explained that both she and her granddaughter were distraught at the thought of her losing her purple hair. This lady was known for her purple hair – it was part of her identity and had been for many years. Her granddaughter felt that her grandma would not be the same person without it. Luckily, a local hairdresser was able to put colour through the wig. An identity was maintained.

I meet a lot of women who wear wigs. I can honestly say that if I do realise that they are wearing a wig, it is for one of two reasons:

1. They tell me.
2. They keep fiddling with the wig, moving and readjusting it.

My advice is to get your wig fitted by a professional; practise putting it on and then forget about it. No one knows, unless you want them to know.

Looking After Your Wig

It was a surprise to me that wigs need washing. Not only do they need washing, but different types of wig, human hair and fibre-based systems, require washing at different times.

Your wig needs to be washed when the hair doesn't move as it once did and the colour becomes flat. In Audrey's experience, fibre wigs tend to need washing at least once every four weeks. Human hair usually needs washing every two weeks.

Specialist shampoos and conditioners and stay-in conditioners should always be used, and your consultant will be able to advise you. See Appendix 3 for some detailed instructions.

Refreshing Your Wig

As your wig is next to your scalp for long periods of time, you might want to 'refresh' your wig in between washes. I suggest a daily spritz with a natural antibacterial solution, such as tea tree floral water. Spray onto the inside of your wig and leave to dry.

There is no item of clothing that you would leave next to your skin every day for weeks before you wash it. I understand that washing a wig too often can damage it and shorten its useful life. I'll leave it to your wig specialist to tell you about washing, but please consider refreshing it at least every evening. It will be beneficial to your scalp health and may well result in fewer breakouts.

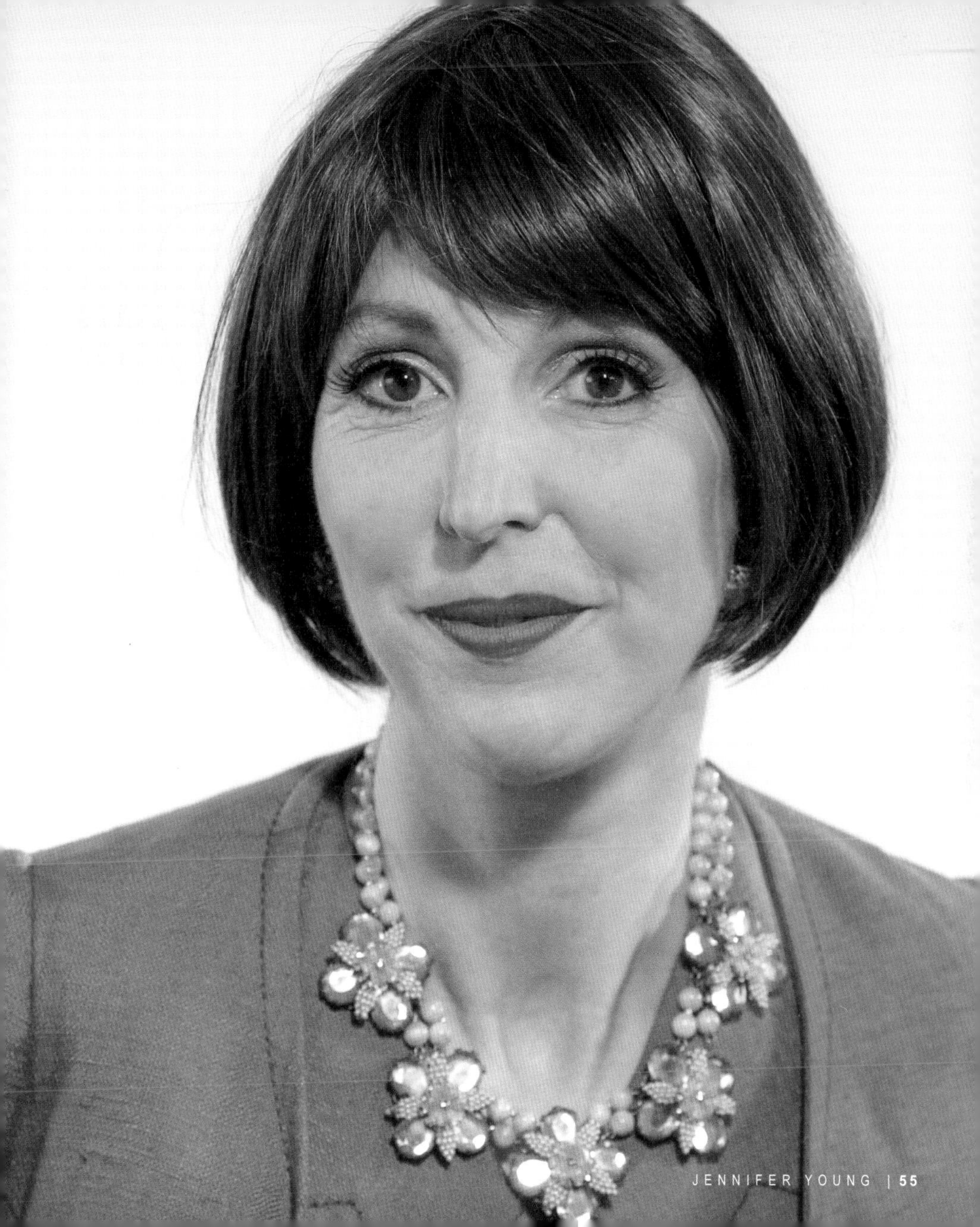

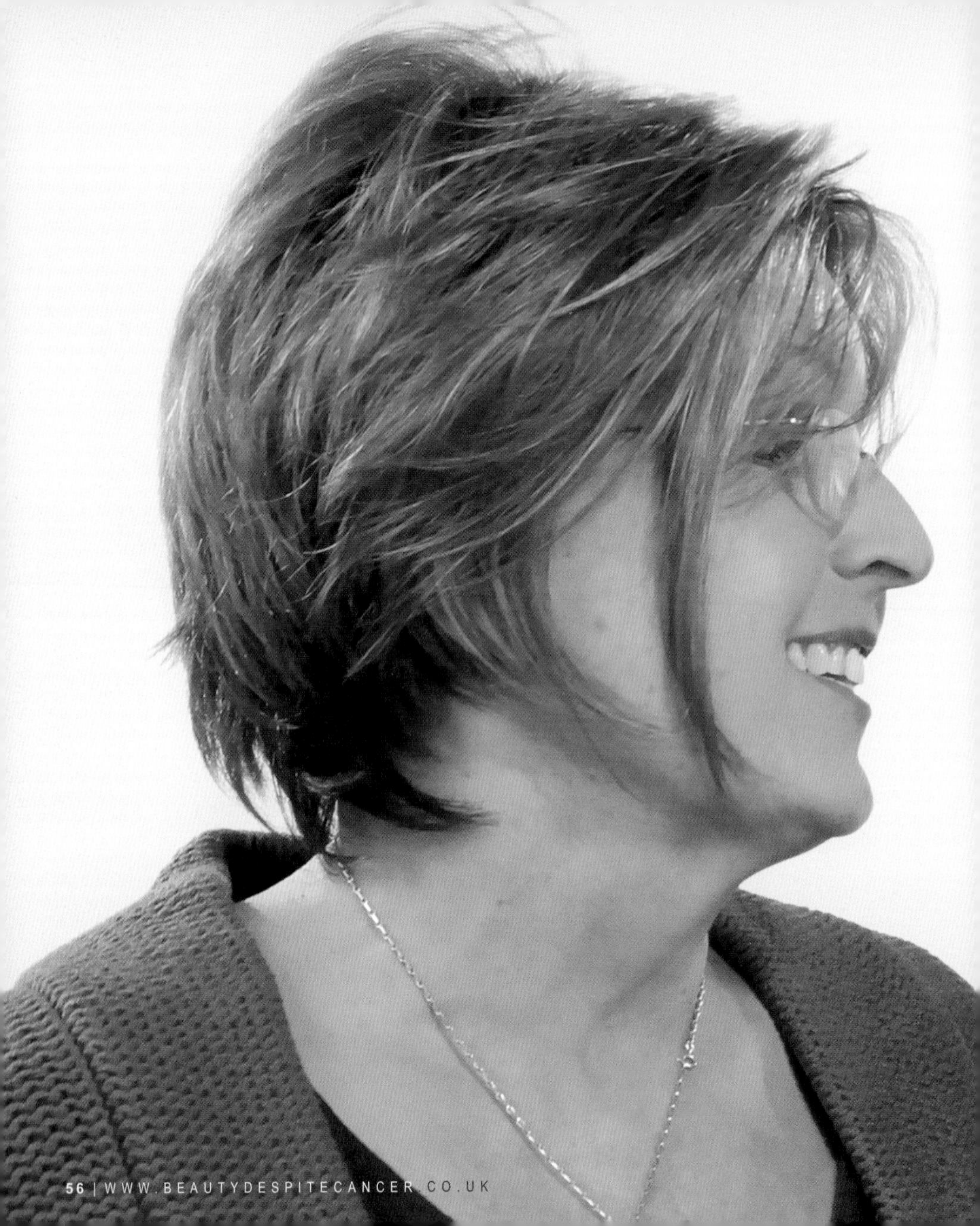

Fitting your wig

Make sure your wig fits – it can be altered

Place on or above your hairline (four fingers above your eyebrows)

A fringe can camouflage lost eyebrows

Use highlights and let the roots show

Layers create movement

Finger comb to create a natural look

Accessorise with a scarf or jewellery or create a messy up-style

Use the right brush

Don't fiddle with your wig – forget about it

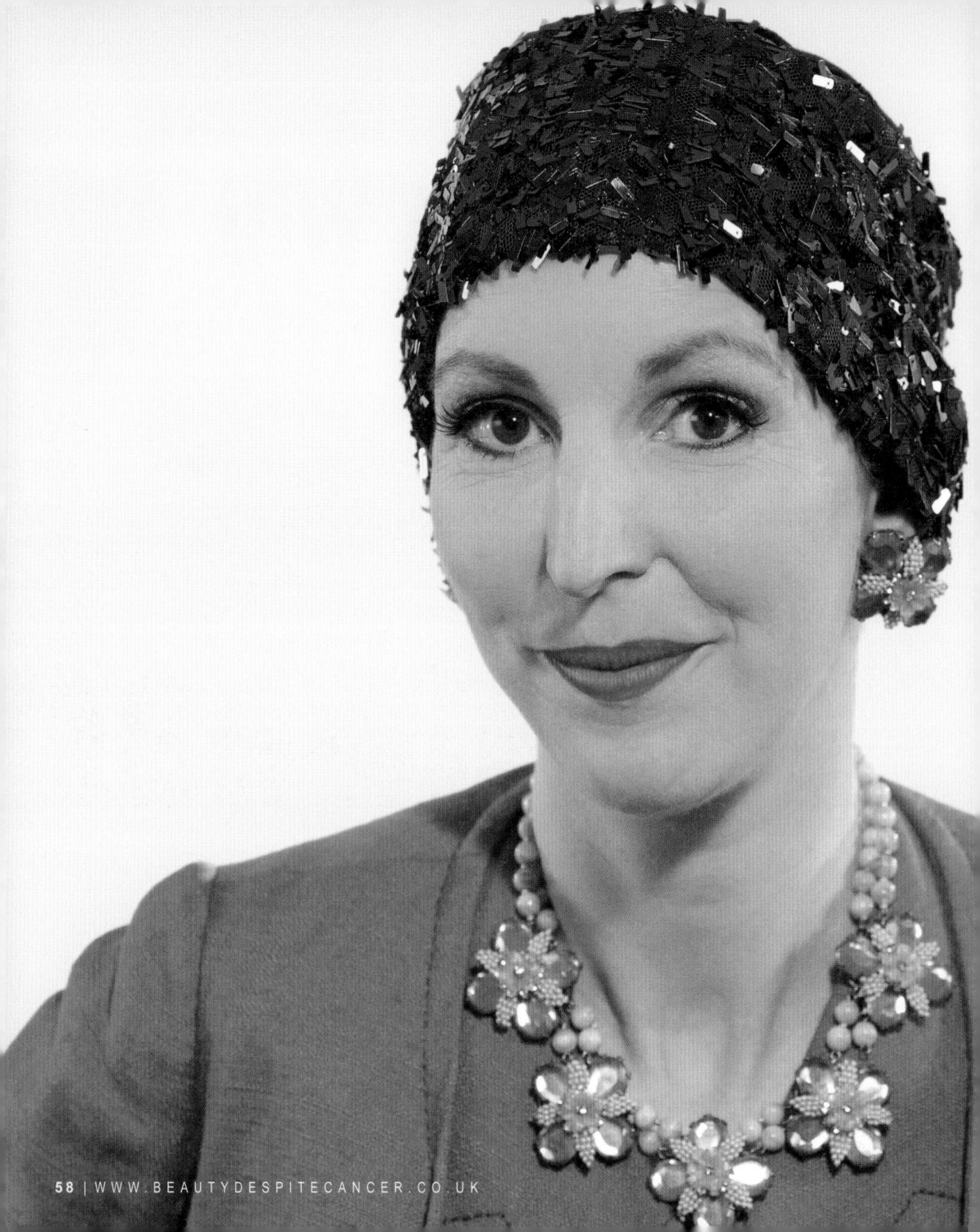

Headwear

Alternatives to Wigs

Wigs can be hot and uncomfortable. I know lots of ladies who save them for special occasions or who wear them for the school run, as their children prefer them to do so. There are, however, some more-comfortable options available to you.

Hairpieces

Hairpieces are so realistic that we decided not to use them for the shoot. The one we tried looked too much like a hat with hair underneath.

The images for this book have to be clear about what they portray: the beauty of a woman without hair, a wig (which cannot be identified as such) or a stylish head cover.

The hairpiece under a hat confused us all and we knew what we were looking for. A hairpiece is as effective as a wig in helping one to look as though one has a full head of hair but is a lot cooler. It is also a less expensive option.

Again, your wig fitter can help; ask about fringe pieces or pony tails, both to wear under a hat or scarf.

Scarves and Hats

'I don't wear my wig in the house. I keep a soft beany next to the front door so that I am not caught out when I have a delivery or when the window cleaner calls.'

Caron, The Wirral

There is a wide range of styles and colours designed for those living with hair loss. Specialist manufacturers work exclusively with those experiencing medical hair loss. There are comfortable styles available for all occasions, seasonal options to ensure comfort and coolness, swimming caps, and sleeping hats.

Most suppliers provide you with an information sheet to demonstrate how a particular item can be worn, sometimes supporting this with video instruction. Your wig fitter will have the training and experience to demonstrate how to fit and use a scarf.

Scarves can be tricky to fit; they are certainly more difficult to wear than a hat. It is important to be comfortable and confident with your scarf. Don't allow yourself to be in the same position as Beauty Despite Cancer writer Sam

Reynolds. Sam is a self-taught expert in tying scarves – she spent hours in the changing room of a well-known high street store learning her craft soon after she lost her hair to chemo. It was one of the loneliest experiences of her treatment. I caution against it.

Choosing the Right Headwear

How do you decide upon a hat or a scarf? How do you know what suits you and which hat goes best with which outfit? This is uncharted territory for many.

I wouldn't know where to start, so I asked Claire Featherstone, our Beauty Despite Cancer 'chemo headwear' expert and headwear stylist for our photo shoot. Claire advises her clients to take a number of factors into consideration:

- Season
- Style
- Function
- Colour
- Complexion

Season

Season is the first thing to think about. The time of year in which your treatment starts could dictate the type of fabric that you want for your headwear. If it is spring or summer and you envisage needing to keep cool, choose something that is unlined and made of cotton, for example.

The opposite is true in winter. You can lose lots of body heat through your head, so wrap up warm.

Style and Function

The style decision is personal: some of us prefer a casual look (a stretch jersey-style hat) and others like to be more formal (a silk headscarf). Remember that you might want a head cover that is an ‘everyday throw-on’.

Many ladies wear a neck scarf, as this area can feel exposed when not covered by hair.

Colour

This is easiest to decide upon when you look at the contents of your wardrobe. If you wear a lot of print, then choose a plain fabric; if your wardrobe is very plain, then choose a print.

If your throw-on is for dog walking and it is winter, match (or clash) with your winter coat.

Choosing your headwear for work can be trickier, but the same rules apply. If you wear a uniform, consider its colour when making your decision.

Complexion

Next, consider your skin tone and eye colour. Pick a blue, green, grey or brown print to highlight your eye colour.

Be careful that the colour you choose to match your favourite outfit doesn't make you look 'washed out'. You can find some colour-matching advice in the 'Style' section in Chapter 3.

Make-up is important too (Chapter 2). You might need to apply more when going through chemo, and if you know you are going to wear, for example, bright red lipstick, then pick a red headscarf or hat.

The Look

When you have chosen your headwear, experiment. Do your ears look better tucked in or out? Try some big earrings. Pull together some looks that work with your wardrobe and make you feel confident.

Ask a friend to help by taking photos of several different outfits with a headscarf, shoes and a bag. Stick the photos onto the inside of your wardrobe door so that you don't have to think about anything when you get dressed.

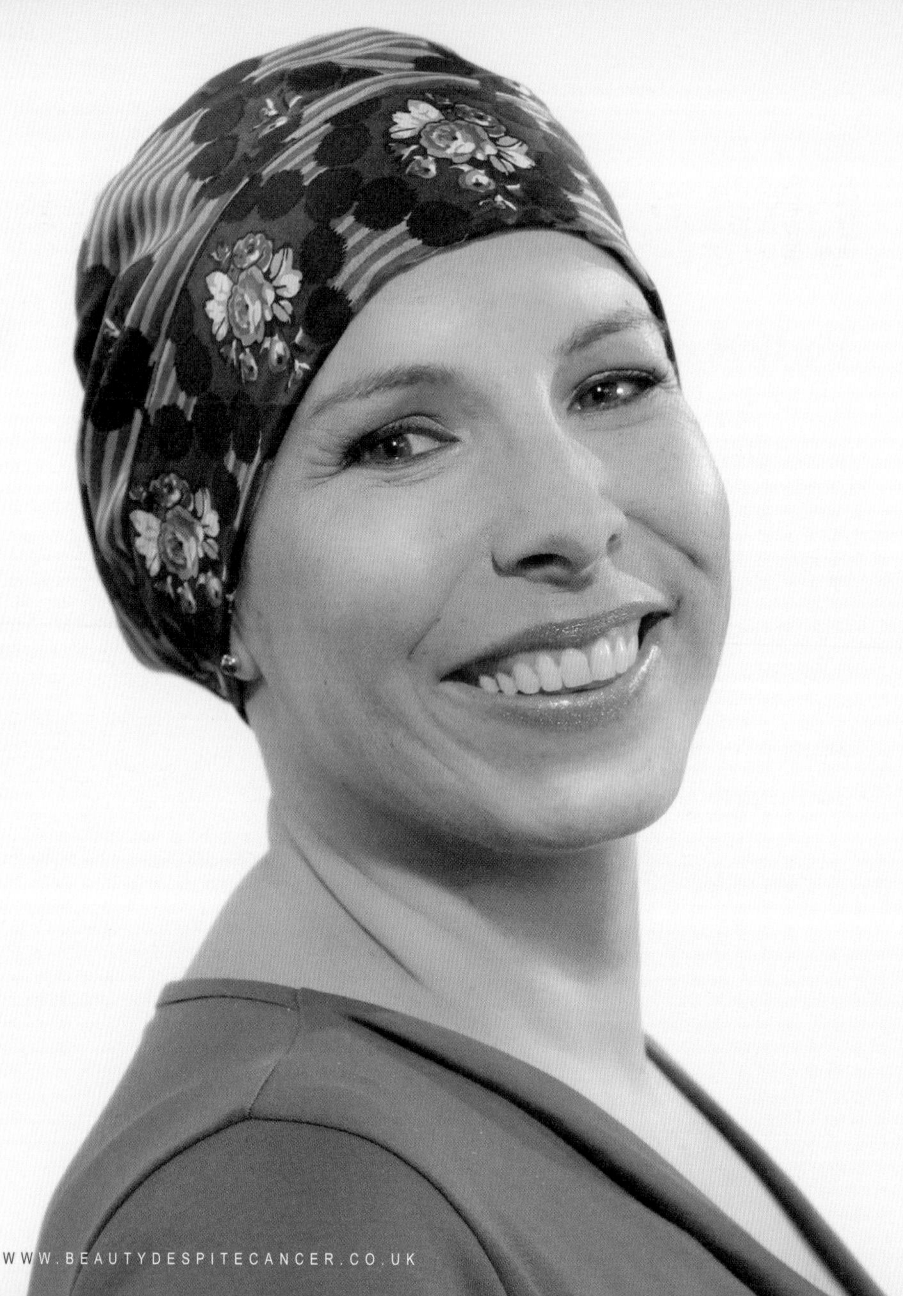

Choosing headwear

Colour – choose a colour that makes you look fabulous and matches your outfit, shoes, nails or lipstick

Fabric– let the season determine the material

Function – do you need a headscarf to wear as you walk the dog or a party scarf?

Complexion – keep your complexion in mind, it will determine the colour and style of your headwear

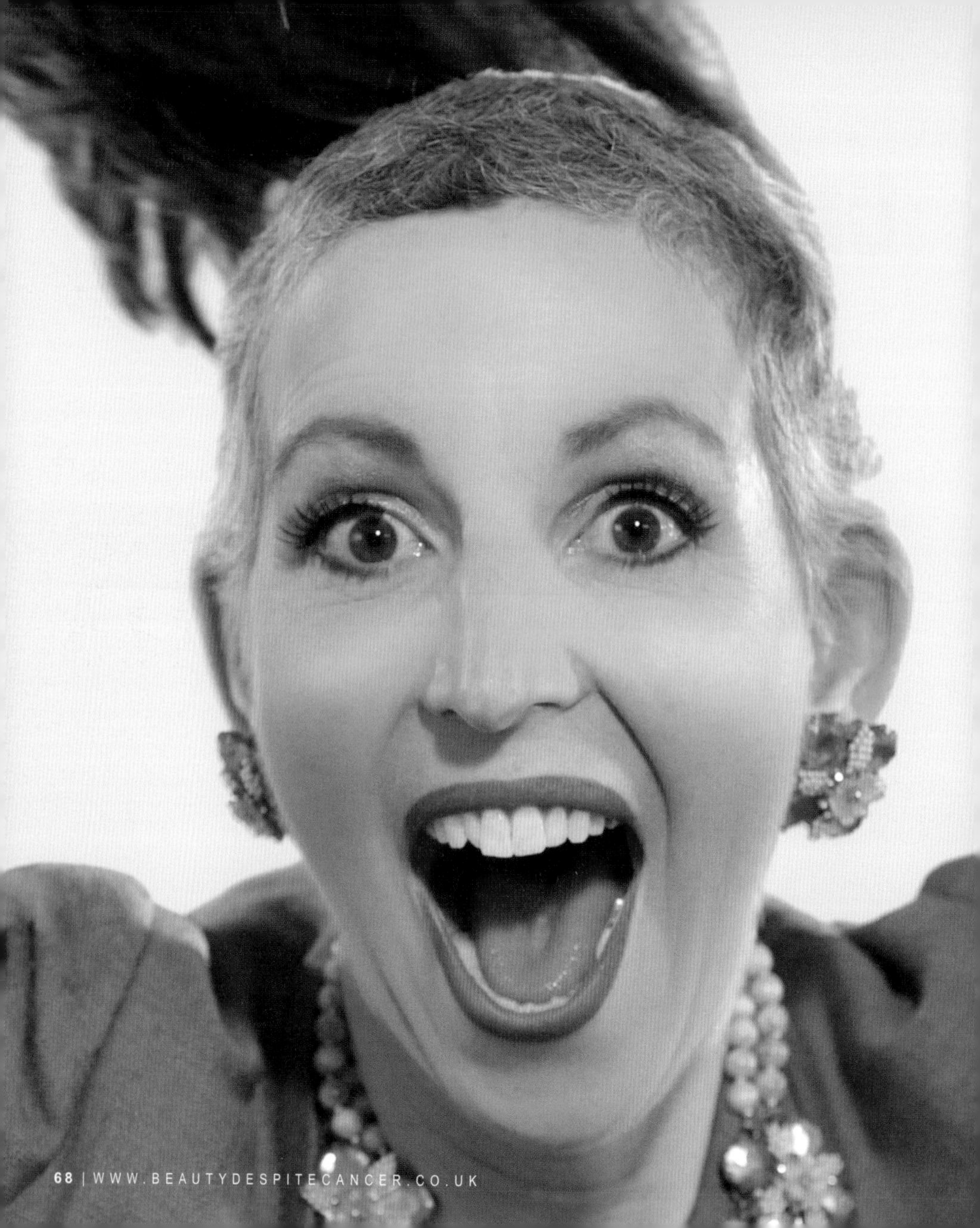

Regrowth

Regrowth

'When hair grows again it can be a different colour or texture or change from curly or straight. The regrowth often reverts to your usual hair in time. These changes result when chemotherapy alters the shape and size of the follicles and therefore of the hair shafts that grow from the follicles. Altered melanin production affects the colour.'

Sara Allison, Trichologist

Any hair lost to chemotherapy will grow back. It might take a while but it will come back. Trichologist Sara Allison, an expert in hair and scalp disorders, tells us that you can expect regrowth three to four months after treatment ends, but the new hair might not be the same as your pre-treatment hair.

When regrowth begins, it is the time to embrace change. Maximiliano Centini considers four main elements when styling hair as it returns:

- Hair type
- Face shape
- Lifestyle
- Figure

Max tailors his cut accordingly. He recommends a pixie cut, as it suits everyone when the four key elements are taken into account and influence the styling.

If you are keen to get your long hair back, the transition is easier than you might think, as long as you have a plan. Max manages hair growth for his clients. He starts by keeping the sides and back shorter, allowing the top to grow. The hair looks neat and styled, and the silhouette is flattering to all face shapes.

As the top grows down onto the sides of the face, Max adds layers to the top, giving volume. The nape area is kept shorter until the length reaches the hairline.

'I am never going to have long hair again. My hair used to reach my waist. I was horrified at the thought of losing it. I would never have had short hair by choice. Now, I am never going back to long. Short suits me and it is a lot easier to manage.'

Cathy, Staffordshire

Hair Colouring

Everyone I meet is advised against colouring their hair during treatment and when it begins to grow back.

When you are able to colour your hair again, both it and you might have changed. Many of the women I speak to are reluctant to return to the hair colours that they used previously, now preferring a more natural colouring system. Trichologist Sara Allison also believes that a natural hair colour is more appropriate at this stage of regrowth.

There are a lot of natural dyes to choose from: some colour the hair by penetrating the hair shaft, some do not. Those, such as henna, that do not penetrate the hair shaft will wash away with time.

There are several factors to take into account when deciding upon your hair colour.

If natural isn't important to you:

- You can do what you used to do – visit your hairdresser or buy your old home colour, making sure that a patch test and a strand test are done.

If you prefer natural:

- Are you happy to have a colour that will fade with time and after washes?
- Are you prepared for a long and not particularly glamorous colouring session?

If your answers to these last two questions are 'yes' and your hair is dark, then henna is for you.

Henna is completely natural. Read the ingredients label on the product you choose, to make sure that the manufacturer hasn't added any chemicals. If the product contains additives, keep looking until you find one that is natural.

'We advise our patients not to colour their hair during treatment, as it can block the follicles. Their bodies have enough to contend with without adding hair colour to it. The less that is done to new hair the better, as it is very fragile'

Alina, Clinical Nurse Specialist – Breast Care, Elstree Cancer Centre

Ask the henna salesperson for advice about the colour to use.

Be warned, henna smells bad and it takes a long time to colour your hair. Henna needs reapplying more frequently than other hair colours, as it isn't a dye and doesn't penetrate the hair shaft. It will cover grey hair, but all the grey hairs will have a lighter henna colour than your non-grey hairs.

A patch test and strand test are necessary. When you are sure you don't react to the henna, off you go.

How to apply henna:

- Follow the mixing instructions that accompany the henna product.
- Apply a barrier cream just underneath your hairline, over your ears and to your hands (if you are applying the henna).
- Divide your hair into sections and use a dye applicator brush to apply the henna to the hair, starting at the roots and moving towards the ends.

'The more natural the hair dye, the less likely there will be a reaction and associated breakage or shedding. I suggest a semi-permanent or temporary dye. Make sure your hairdresser does a strand test, as dye may take differently on your new hair. After about six months, your hair and scalp may be resilient enough for you to be able to revert to permanent dyes.'

Sara Allison, Trichologist

- When all your hair is covered with henna, place a plastic bag over it. The bag should contain your hair and the henna.
- Fasten the plastic bag with a knot or twist at the front or side of your head.
- Cover the bag with a towel, just as you would when your hair is wet from washing.
- Wait three hours – yes, three hours! The depth of your colour is determined by the length of time that the henna remains on your hair. You can wait for a mere two hours if you wish. There have been occasions when I have left mine on for longer than three hours. Experiment and see what difference the length of time makes to your colour.
- When your waiting time is up, wash your hair to remove the henna. Be warned, this is messy and your hair will need a couple of washes. I always use conditioner first to take away most of the henna, then wash, then condition again and, finally, wash.

- Henna will continue to wash from your hair. Don't panic, as I did, if the water in your first post-henna bath is orange – it is the henna, not you!
- If you don't dry your hair immediately, protect fabrics from it – the colour will 'leak' from your wet hair and will stain anything that it comes into contact with. Pillows have been ruined in this way.

I know! That was the stuff of your teens and now you enjoy a cup of tea with the hairdresser who has lovingly cared for your hair for the last 20 years. Don't despair – talk to your hairdresser about natural salon colours, of which there are many and some that are organic.

FACE

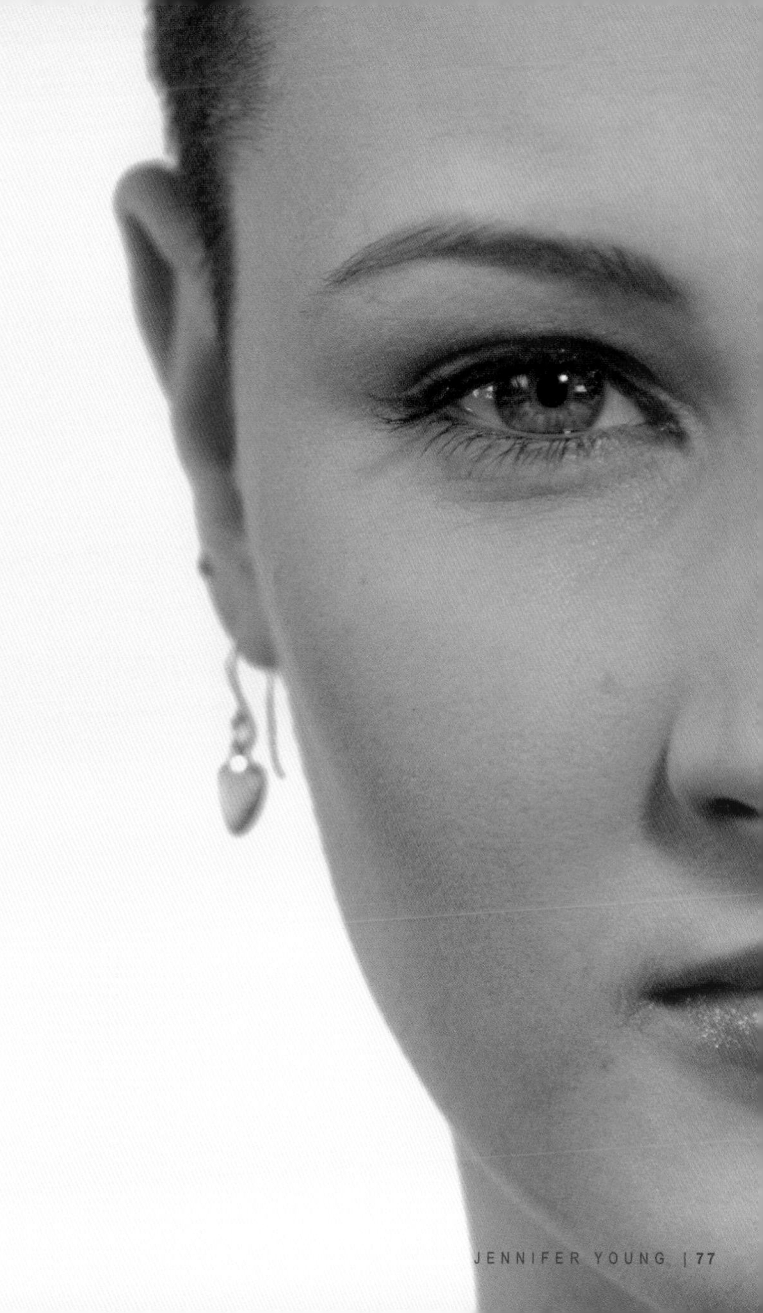

Caring for Your Face

'I can't go out looking like this.'

Caller to Beauty
Despite Cancer Appearance Advice Line

For some, treatment has no impact on appearance, while for others, it is distinct and traumatic. If you feel significantly changed, it may be a challenge for you to have the confidence to 'face the world'.

Let's take it one step at time and, having dealt with hair in the last chapter, we will now look after your skin and then work our way downwards, from the eyes to the lips.

Anti-ageing

The concept of ageing can trigger conflicting emotions. Many tell me that they feel lucky every birthday, but they still don't want to look old.

I often ask patients what they would like their

skincare products to do for them – 'make me look younger' is usually the top answer.

There are many reasons why cancer treatment could 'ravage' you. The following list was drawn up by some ladies at Cancer Support Scotland in Glasgow:

- Worry[6]
- Anxiety[6]
- Lack of sleep
- Premature menopause (part of the treatment for many cancers)
- Hospital environment (heating or air conditioning)
- Poor nutrition, as a result of low appetite
- A craving for sugar when fatigued
- Stress[6]
- Depression[6]
- Fatigue[7]

It's OK to want to look like you, and there are many things that you can do to combat the signs of ageing, both during and after treatment, if that is your wish. Here are my top five suggestions for managing ageing as you go through treatment.

Skincare

'Cancer treatment has ravaged me and aged me beyond my years.

Nothing has aged me as cancer has aged me.'

Fiona, Wales

Caring for your skin is probably the easiest of all of my anti-ageing suggestions. Following a skincare routine (see 'Skincare Routine' section in this chapter) can counteract the environmental stresses placed upon your skin. It will also give you something to focus on, other than the things that may be worrying you. Skincare is very therapeutic as well as being enjoyable. It is a treat with benefits.

Complementary Therapies

Research has shown that complementary therapies can significantly reduce anxiety in cancer patients[7], lowering the likelihood of depression.[8-14]Taking away one of the 'drivers' of ageing can only be good.

Please take a look at Appendix 4 before choosing your therapist.

Sleep

Around 75% of people with cancer suffer from some kind of fatigue. Some hospitals even offer 'fatigue groups'[7], such is the importance of sleep.

I am a huge fan of sleep and a big believer in 'beauty sleep'. Research[15] has found that those deprived of sleep are rated as less attractive than those who have had a good eight hours. If nothing else can motivate you to get to bed early, then this should!

Sleeping is difficult when there are so many things to worry about. It will help on so many levels. Pat Duckworth, Harley Street Master NLP Practitioner and cognitive hypnotherapist, shares her sleep tips in Appendix 5. You might not find them easy at first. It is worth investing in your sleep – there are so many benefits, not all of which are beauty related.[15-17]

Appetite and Nutrition

Feeding the skin from the inside is just as important as feeding the skin from the outside. Your appetite may be reduced at times, but when you feel able to eat, consider eating well. I think we've all experienced the need to reach for sugar, be it in the form of alcohol, chocolate or cake, when we are tired. If that's what you need to do, by all means do it and don't even consider feeling anything but joy about the choice you have made.

If you are concerned about eating well during your treatment, think about consulting a specialist nutritional therapist, or an oncology dietician. If that's not an option for you, Appendix 6 has some examples of recipes that are great for skin health and anti-ageing.

Hormones

If your hormones are being controlled as part of your treatment, it is for a good reason. Your medical team will have explained their reasoning to you, so there's no need for me to go over it all again.

The hormone oestrogen is implicated in the growth of many cancers. Unfortunately, it is also a 'youthful' hormone – lowered levels can affect nails, skin and hair.

The medical team that I worked with in order to create the Defiant Beauty Collections, and others that I have since met, routinely advise their patients to avoid oestrogenic ingredients in their skincare and cosmetics. I was specifically asked not to include natural oestrogens in the skincare collections that I created for use by cancer patients.

Some medical teams, on the other hand, suggest that oestrogenic substances are a solution to some of the skin damage caused by cancer treatments.

I can't answer this dilemma for you, as medical opinion varies. All I can say is that non-oestrogenic ingredients exist that have potent anti-ageing effects and there is no need to use products that contain oestrogens, natural or otherwise.

Skincare

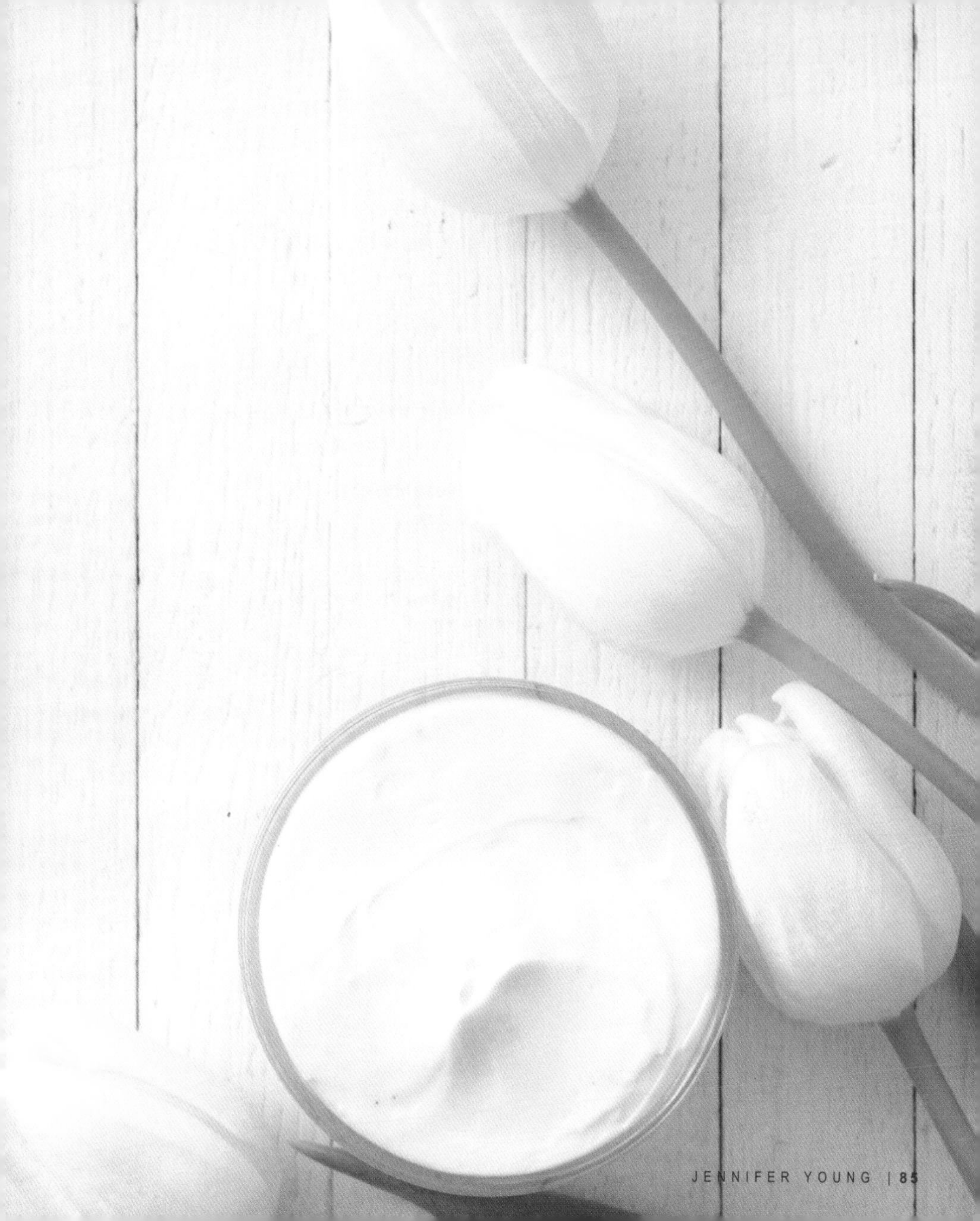

Skincare Routine

A skincare routine is now even more important than usual. Most people need to prepare their skin for make-up – a skincare routine is that preparation. Don't skip straight to make-up; build the foundation first.

The following skincare routine is an excellent base for the application of your cosmetics. You may not have had a regime before: if you feel unable to do too much for your skin, prioritise, and do only this.

Cleansing

Every stage of a skincare routine is important, but cleansing is the one that is often neglected. 'Chemo skin' needs some looking after, as it is so sensitive and can be sore.

Find a cleansing balm. Balms are simple products that are moisturising as well as cleansing. Follow the directions on the product. Most balms can be used as a facemask as well as a cleanser.

Use it first as a cleanser: apply to the face and wipe away using cotton wool. Reapply as a mask and cover with hot cotton cloths or lie in a warm bath while wearing the mask. Remove using the cotton cloths or cotton wool.

I always recommend a double cleanse; if you don't have time to use the balm as a mask (keeping it on for longer before removing), reapply after the first cleanse and remove with cotton wool.

Boil your cotton cloths and sponges after use. Your immunity is low and you should prevent your exposure to potentially harmful bacteria that can grow on the damp cotton cloths and sponges.

Exfoliation

Exfoliation is an essential part of a skincare routine, particularly through treatment, as your skin is dry and flaking. However, your skin will also be sore and sensitive, so traditional exfoliators may cause skin damage. Removing your balm with hot cotton cloths has a gentle exfoliating action.

Use your balm and cloths morning and evening, and your skin will be adequately exfoliated. Gentle exfoliating sponges are an alternative to hot cloths.

Toner

I am often asked about the difference between moisturising and hydration, and many wonder how to keep the skin hydrated. I think that hydration comes from within. Keep drinking fluids[18] – water is my favourite. If you need a little help, use a natural facial spritz. Better quality toners and spritzes are leave-on products, and not something for merely removing the last remnants of a cleanser.

By this stage your face should be feeling fabulous! Your skin should be soft from the cleansing balm, smooth from the use of the exfoliating cotton cloths or sponges, and hydrated thanks to the facial spritz.

This might be enough for your skin. If it isn't, it may well be soon. You will be surprised by the change in your skin as you follow your skincare routine. If you still need more, read on…

Facial Oil or Serum

This is the 'must-have' for most of our clients. A serum is an oil-based product for use on the face.

I never recommend creams to those with very sensitive skin (see Appendix 7). An oil is a more intensive moisturising product. Don't use too much. Start by applying a tiny amount and add more if your skin absorbs it. You may find that you need it less and less as your skin's needs change as a result of your new routine.

Karen Stepanova, beauty expert, has some great advice: 'If you want to do only one thing for your skin, use a good cleansing balm morning and evening. Serum is also a good investment. It has a far higher concentration of active ingredients than a moisturiser. The higher concentration makes serum more expensive but means you only need to use a small amount. Serums are capable of penetrating the skin to a deeper level and are used to treat dehydration or dryness. They are a must in everyone's skincare routine.'

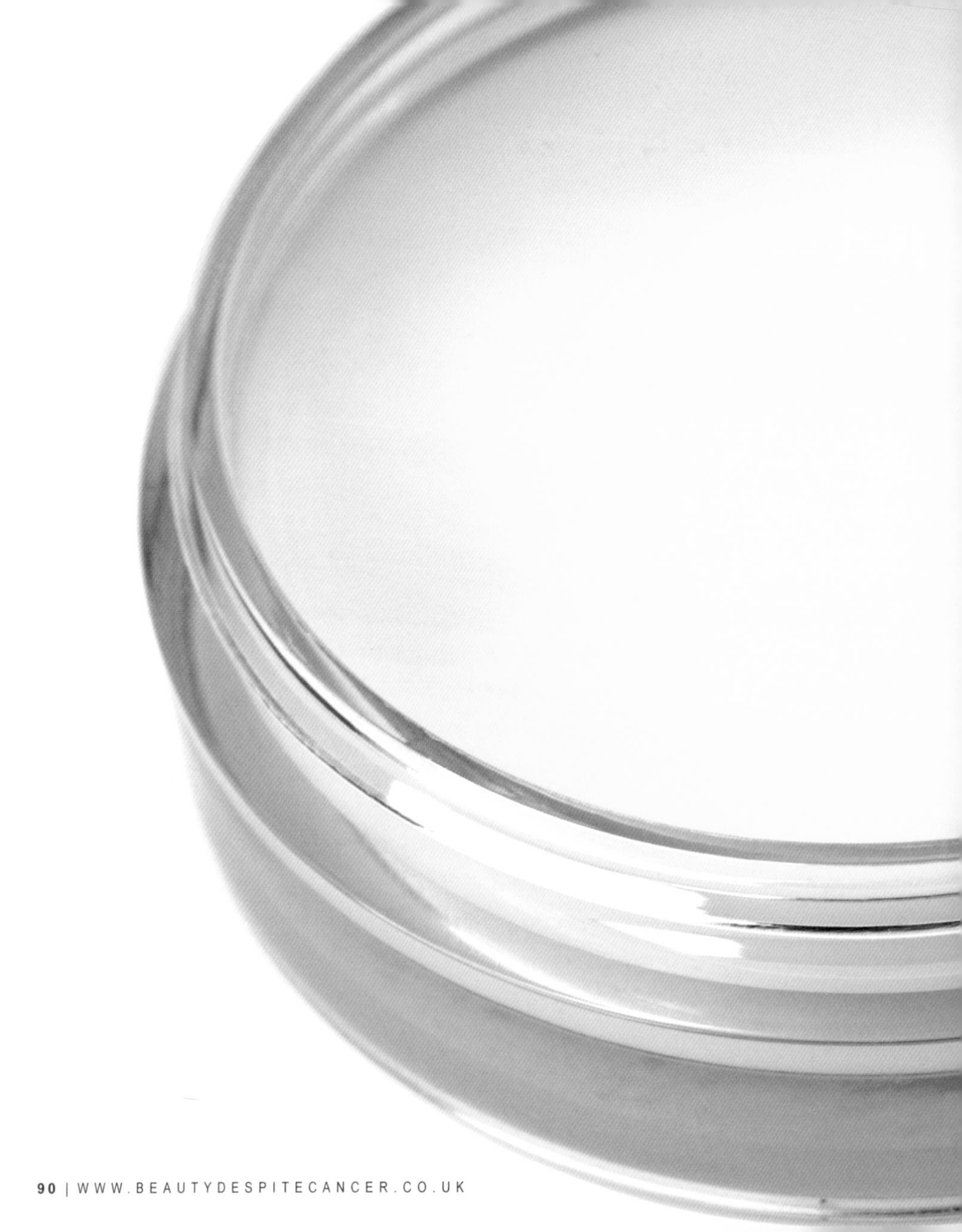

Choosing Skincare

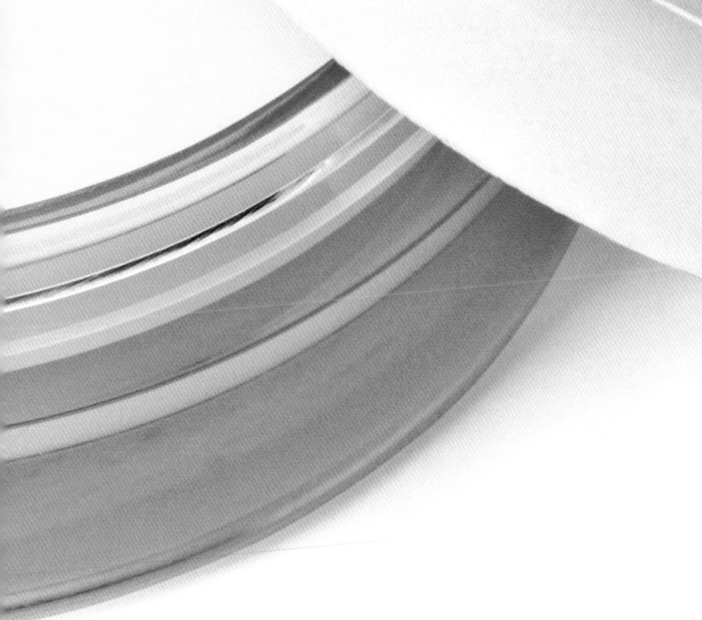

Choosing Your Skincare Products

You may find that your values change as you go through treatment and you now prefer something more 'natural' than your previous choices. Whatever your preferences and values, the steps to choosing the perfect skincare are the same.

What Do You Want to Achieve?

The first and most important step is deciding what you want from your skincare. Usually we are offered a choice of products according to a skin type – dry, oily, etc.

It is important to know your skin type, but you will get more from your products if you turn this approach on its head. Start by asking yourself: 'What do I want my skincare to achieve?'

Most of us have anti-ageing on the list, along with our skin type. Ask for more. Would you like the ingredients in your product to promote sleep, to enhance its anti-ageing effect? Are age spots an additional concern? At first it may be difficult to create your list, because you are used to being offered a limited number of choices – persevere, soon it will be fun.

Next, discover the ingredients that match your needs. Many natural ingredients have specific properties. For example, jojoba oil is great for combination skin (skin that has both oily and dry patches).

Many natural products are fragranced with essential oils, all of which have therapeutic properties as well as a nice smell. Look for orange blossom in the ingredients list if you want help with sleeping. If you want something more stimulating, however, orange blossom is the last thing you need!

Appendix 8 shows you how to read an ingredients label on skincare products sold in the EU.

Fragrance

Chemotherapy can make you nauseous, and sometimes certain smells can trigger that nausea. If you prefer a fragrance-free product, add that to your list.

Essential Oils

The essential oils used for fragrance in natural products contain 'sensitisers'. These are natural constituents of essential oils, but their natural origin does not make them any less irritating to your skin if you have a sensitivity.

The only way to find out is to try products that contain essential oils. You can patch test other ingredients, but don't put undiluted essential oils directly on to your skin.

Very Sensitive Skin

I always advise clients with very sensitive skin to avoid products containing essential oils and to choose products that contain no more than five ingredients. The more ingredients there are in a product, the greater the chance of a skin reaction.

Go Shopping

When you have your wish list, hit the shops. Ask lots of questions of the person selling the products. You can describe your needs without giving away your medical history. If your skin has been affected by your treatment, describe it as very sensitive, dry, sore and reactive. There is no need to mention why this is the case, unless you want to.

If the sales assistant doesn't know the products at an ingredient level and is unable to tell you which ingredients provide which benefits, move on. You deserve to buy your skincare from a specialist. This doesn't mean that you are doomed to buy expensive products. I have asked questions of sales assistants for some very expensive brands and they have no clue as to the ingredients, let alone the benefits.

You are special – buy your skincare from a specialist.

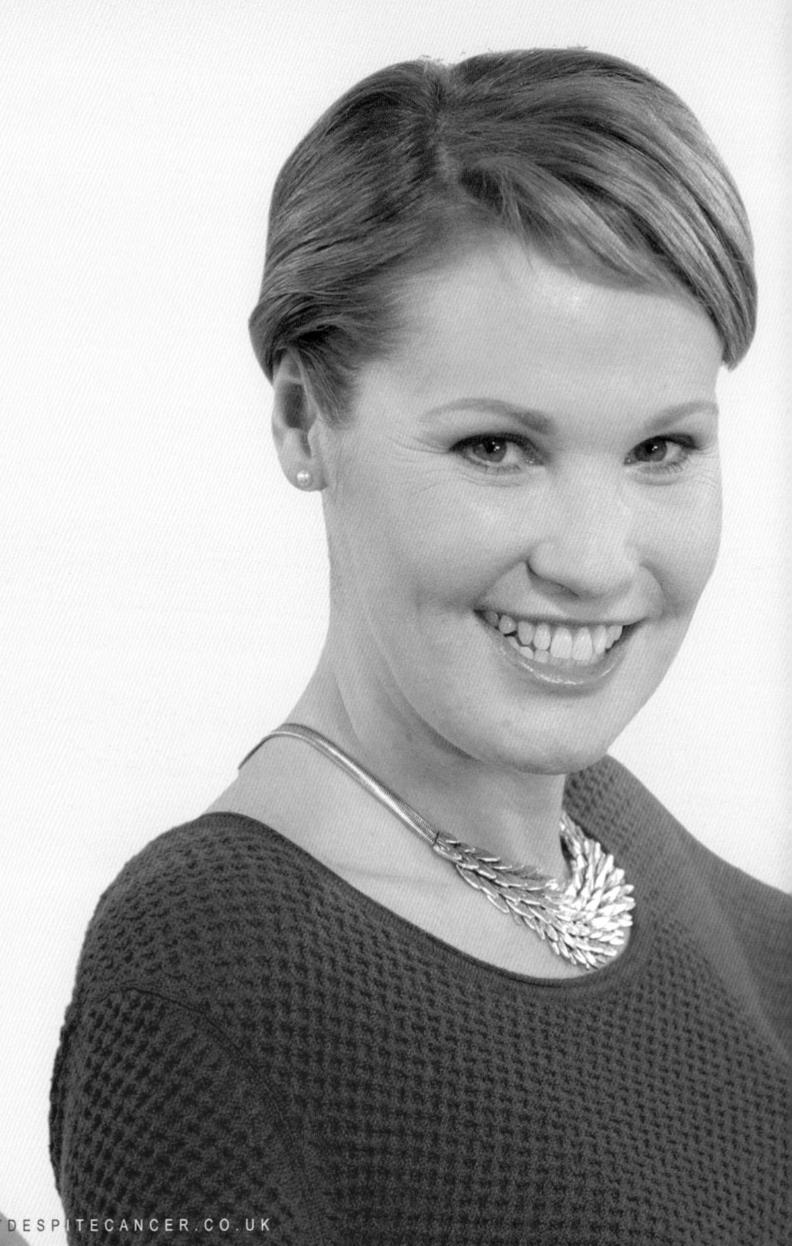

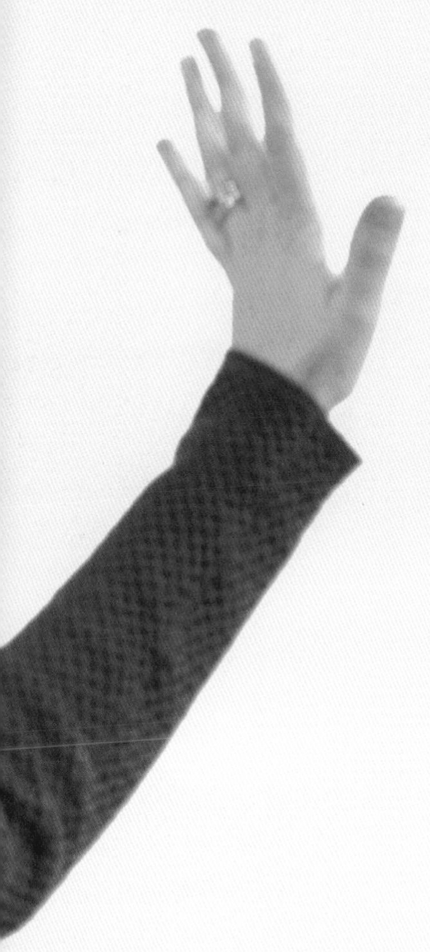

Eyes

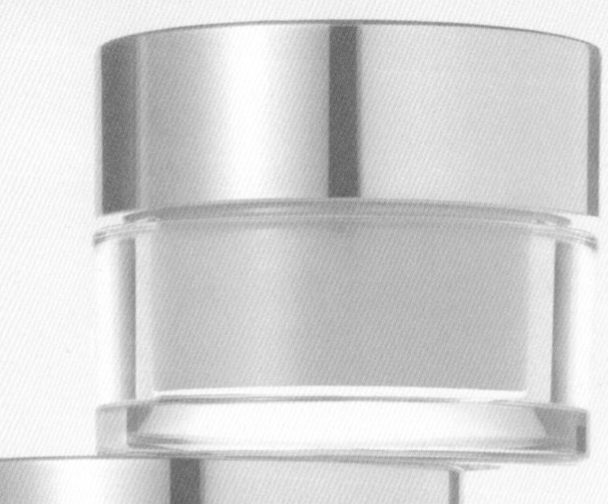

The statistics speak for all of us. In 2014, an estimated one million women in the UK used eye make-up more than once a day.[19]

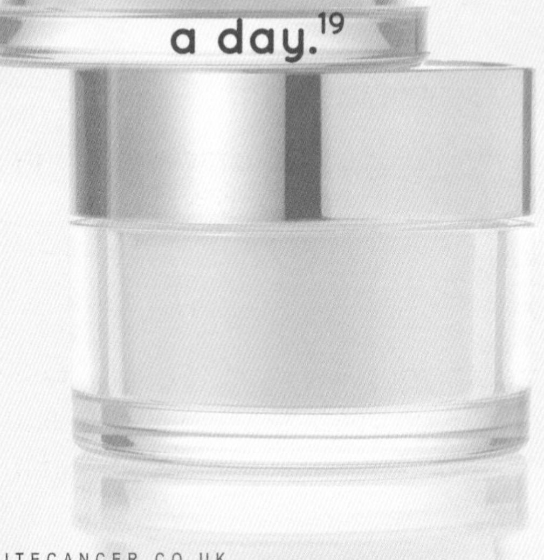

Eyes

The hair loss caused by some chemotherapy regimes can result in sparse eyebrows and lashes. Forewarned is forearmed – there are many ways of recreating your brows and giving the impression of lashes.

Eyebrows

Preparation

If you are reading this before treatment, take a picture of your brows. If you don't like your brows as they are, use a pencil to amend your photo and design your new brows.

Replacing your eyebrows

You have many options – all effective, some expensive and some very simple.

Brush a Brow

You can recreate your whole brow every day, using make-up. Fiona Brunt, a make-up artist working on a chemotherapy ward, suggests a

Brush-a-Brow kit as the most effective way of doing this. A Brush-a-Brow kit usually contains a brow wax, a brow powder and stencils. Louise Boothe, an eyebrow specialist, recommends buying a fine artist's paintbrush (from an art shop) to apply your new brows.

Follow the steps in our Brush-a-Brow guide, remembering to use very fine strokes. It will take some practice. When you have mastered the art, no one will know the brows aren't your own.

You can also use Brush-a-Brow to enhance sparse brows and to thicken thin brows.

I have it on good authority that Sophia Loren shaved her natural eyebrows and recreated them using powder every day. She didn't look too bad, did she?[20]

3D brows

Three-Dimensional brows are, as they say, 3D. Your therapist will recreate an eyebrow that has a third dimension. Most of the 3D brands will attach small synthetic 'hairs' to either your skin or any fine hairs that remain, using an adhesive.

3D brow therapists use various techniques, depending upon the brand with which they have trained. They will use a combination of sculpted paint, eyebrow extensions, tinting and threading to rebuild brows. Remember that photo you took of your brows? Take it with you to the brow salon and a skilled therapist will create your perfect brows.

If you find a good brow technician who specialises in recreating brows where there is no hair, your new brows should last for about two weeks.

The best 3D brow treatments are pure luxury: a facial and a facelift for your eyebrows.

Camouflage

Hide the brow area by putting a fringe into a wig, or by wearing a hairpiece under a hat or scarf. Have your fringe cut so it sits right on your brows. Any longer and it will irritate your eyes, especially if the lashes are thinning.

Cosmetic tattooing

Cosmetic tattooing, also known as semi-permanent make-up, is the longest lasting of all of the eyebrow options. A semi-permanent procedure will last for 12 to 18 months. Needless to say, if it is going to stay for up to 18 months, you want to get your semi-permanents done by a skilled therapist.

First things first – the timing of your procedure is critical. A reputable practitioner won't provide you with semi-permanent brows (or eyeliner to create an illusion of lashes) while you are in treatment. Your immunity is compromised and you are vulnerable to infection.

There is no professional body for cosmetic tattooists. Anyone can practise after completing a short course. It is vital that you decide upon a practitioner with a proven track record and high standards. Many semi-permanent practitioners have experience of medical procedures, such as areola restoration.

I suggest that you ask for a long consultation prior to making an appointment for a treatment and seek reassurance that the practitioner has experience of medical procedures, has very high standards of hygiene and is used to working with those going through treatment or with alopecia clients.

Alopecia clients need individual hair strokes to create the look of a complete brow. If you have a skilled practitioner, you know that when your hair does begin to fall, the tattoo that was behind the eyebrow hair will look realistic and natural.

As this treatment must be carried out prior to your chemotherapy, you don't need to discuss it with your medical team, although they may be able to suggest reputable practitioners.

The pigments used for the tattoo contain iron oxide. You need to tell your medical team about your semi-permanent make-up if you need an MRI before the pigment has been broken down by the body (12–18 months).

I asked Caron Vetter, a semi-permanent make-up practitioner at Whitethorn Fields MediClinic, Stoke Mandeville, to explain why semi-permanent eyebrows are the most popular procedure for cancer patients:

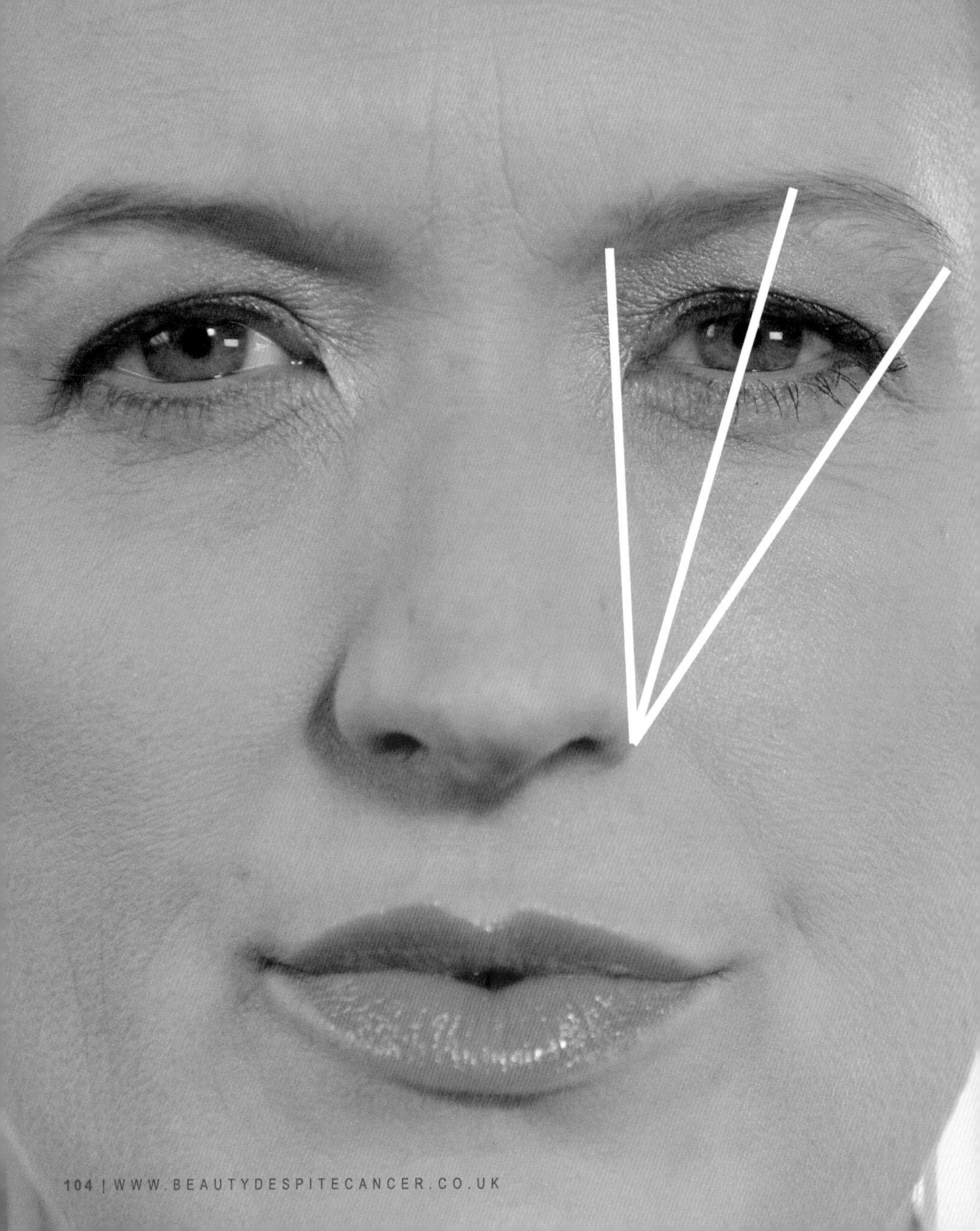

Brow guide

Use your eyebrow pencil or make-up brush to determine where to position your stencil

Hold the brush at the side of your nose, pointing up towards your forehead, passing the outside of your eye; make a mark with your brow powder or pencil

Rotate the pencil, still touching the outside of the nose, until it goes across to the outside edge of your eye; mark the spot–this is where your eyebrow will end

Look straight into the mirror, take the pencil or brush back to the side of your nose. Rotate it so that its line crosses the outside of your pupil; this will be the highest point of your eyebrow

Make a dot slightly higher than first mark as your brow goes up here

Use these marks to position your eyebrow stencil

Using a brush, put a thin layer of wax onto your skin inside the stencil

Use a very thin brush to apply fine strokes to recreate your eyebrows

It takes time to perfect this technique but, once perfected, no one will notice that your brows are your creation.

'Semi-permanent eyebrows can dramatically improve one's self-esteem. As the unpleasant side effects start to take hold, it is one less thing to worry about. You can pick up a mirror and still look like your old self, with all your facial features in place, lifting your appearance!'

Cosmetic tattooing can be used to give an impression of stubble or very short hair. Some men prefer this to wearing a wig.

Eyelashes

Lash illusion

Eyeliner can be used on your eyelid to create an illusion of lashes. This is an incredibly effective technique. No one will notice that your lashes aren't there. I cannot emphasise enough just how effective this technique is – please try it and see for yourself.

'I had some false lashes recently. I felt so feminine, I was fluttering away, it was marvellous. I loved them.'

Audrey, London – she has lived with alopecia for 30 years

Use a full-edge liner brush to apply powder mineral eyeliner to your upper eyelid. Dampen the brush and dip it into the powder. Apply the first strokes to the back of your hand in order to remove excess powder.

Draw a fine, clean line along your top lash line. Extend the line slightly past the corner of your top lash line. Use the same technique to create a line from the middle to the outer edge of your lower lash line.

Eyelash extensions

Please speak to your medical team if you are considering eyelash extensions or false eyelashes. You could be prone to infection:

'Fake eyelashes or eyelash extensions are a necessity. My godmother bought me a session at a local beautician's. I had lashes to be proud of! Once I had lost them all, I used fake eyelashes, and relied on them to make the reflection in the mirror a little more familiar every day.'
Sam Reynolds, Surrey

the eye area is very sensitive and false lashes and extensions can harbour bacteria. If your medical team are happy, read on…

Eyelash extensions are synthetic, usually individual, eyelashes that are applied to the base of your natural lashes using an adhesive. They cannot be applied to an eye that has no eyelashes.

Your extensions will stay only as long as your natural lashes. You may lose your lashes, or some of your lashes, to chemotherapy. Your lash extensions will go with them.

Your therapist can apply a 'bulb' to each of your natural lashes. Each bulb has three lashes on it; if your lashes are sparse, bulbs will make them less so.

False lashes

False lashes can look just as good as extensions and natural lashes. They have the advantage of not requiring natural lashes as an anchoring point. They are removable and are only worn for the day or during an event. This is much more hygienic and more likely to be accepted by your medical team, but you still need to check with them.

If you get the OK, choose natural-looking lashes that add volume not length. Applying false lashes is difficult but not impossible – the more you practise, the better you will become.

Many high-street shops will apply false eyelashes for you when you buy the lashes from them. Some will also apply your eye make-up at the same time. Beware – hygiene standards are variable. If you would like someone else to fix your lashes into position, choose with care (Appendix 4).

False eyelash application

Here's how you can apply the lashes yourself

Cut the lash strips to 1 mm shorter than your eye width

Curl the lashes

Spread lash glue evenly along the back of the strip

Allow the glue to dry until it becomes tacky

Place the lash strip on your eyelid, as close to the natural lash line as possible

Pat into position

Use a matt black eyeliner or eyeshadow to fill any gaps

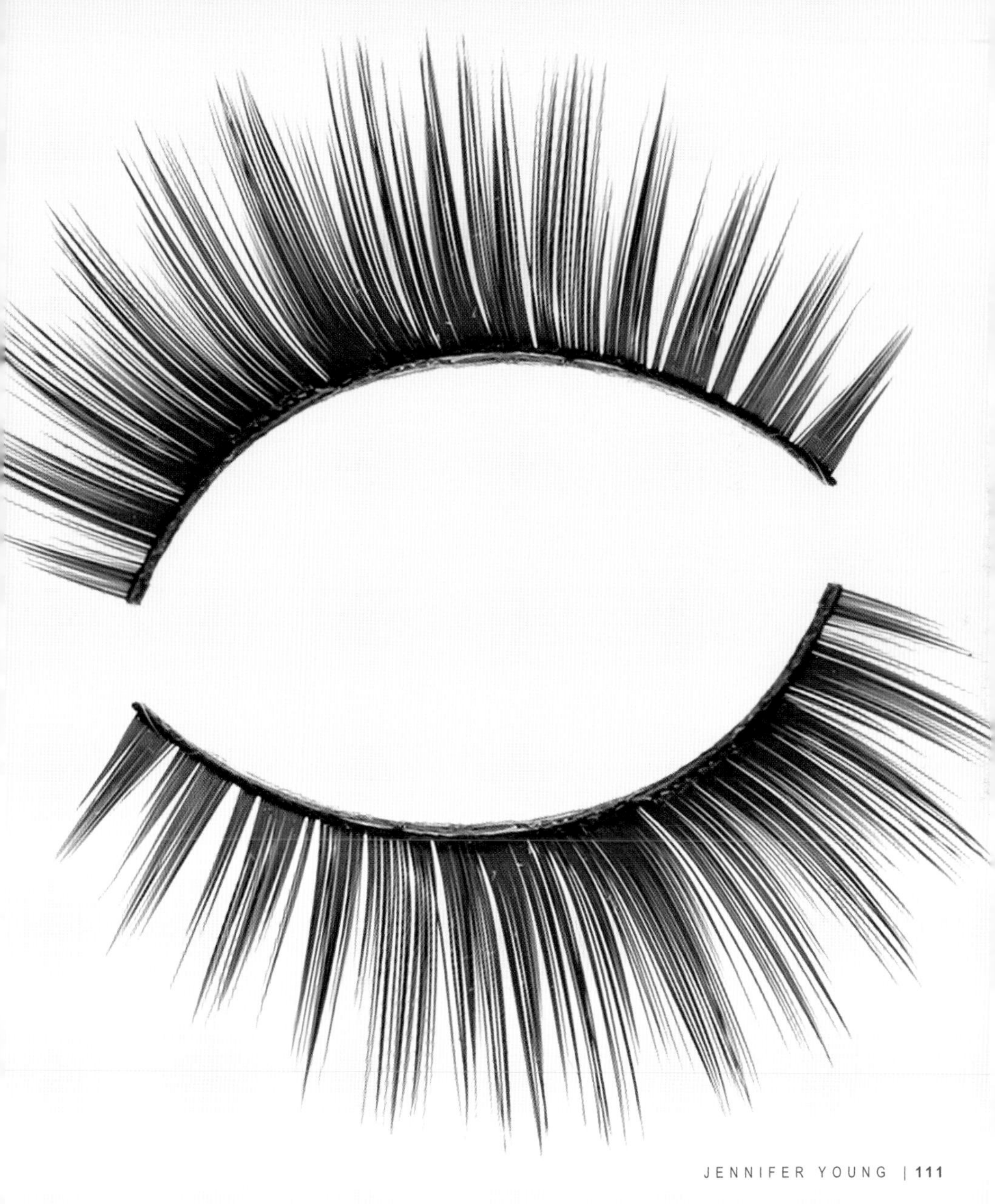

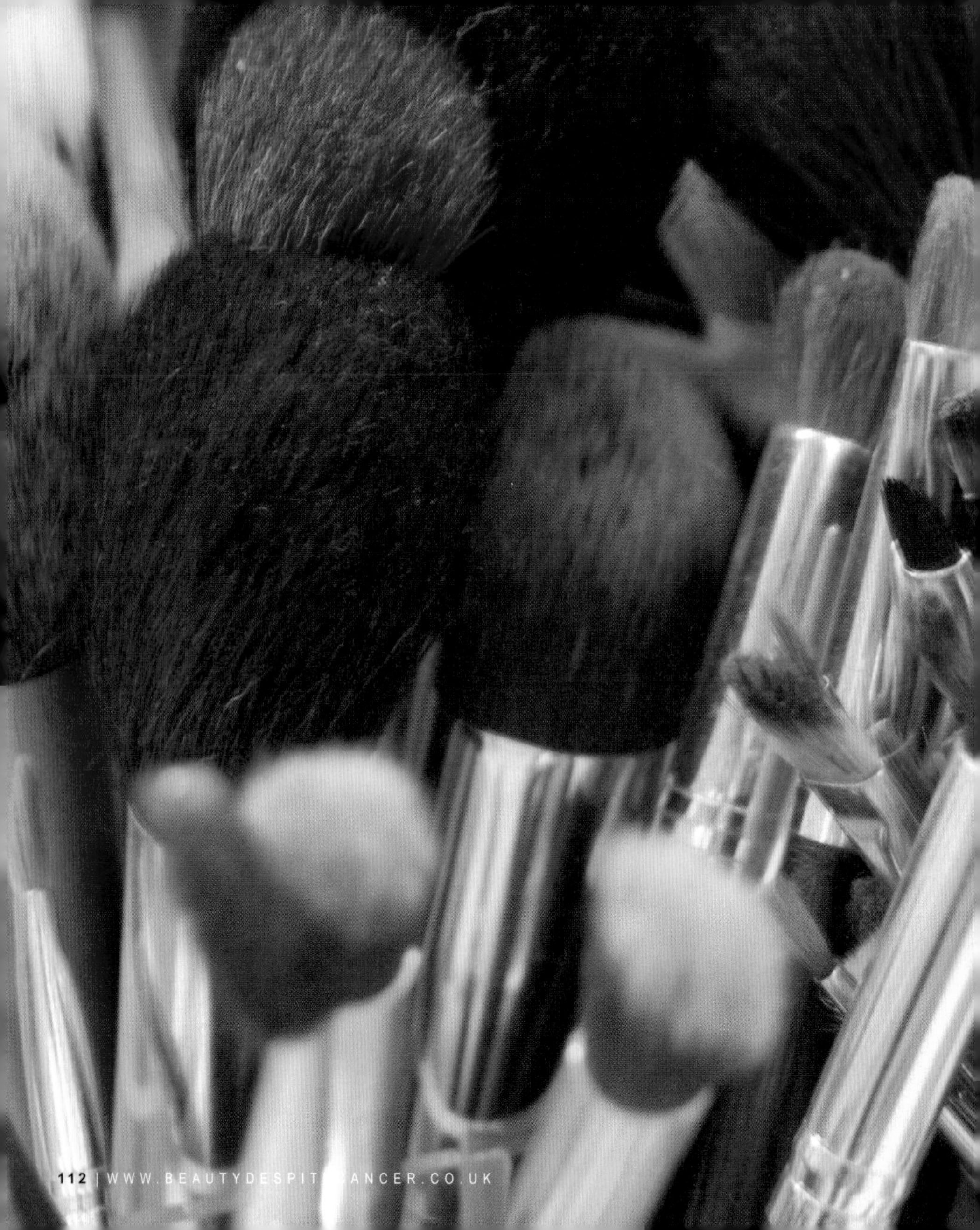

Make-Up

Make-Up

You may well have been applying your make-up for a number of decades. These hints and tips are to help you look more yourself and to provide help in camouflaging some of the common side effects of treatment.

Facial Routine

Provide your make-up with the perfect base by following a skincare routine (see 'Skincare Routine', earlier in this chapter).

Primer

A mineral primer or veil will help to prepare the face for the rest of your make-up. The primer helps to conceal fine lines and to absorb any oils. It will also go some way to normalising skin tone – something that can change as you go through treatment.

Colour correctors

Don't rush into using your foundation. Apply colour correctors if needed. Yellow colour correctors will disguise dark circles around the eyes, green will help to cover ruddy and blemished skin, and blue corrects sallow skin.

Use the colour correctors sparingly, applying them with a brush.

Foundation

Choose a foundation that is very similar to your natural skin tone. I recommend a natural mineral foundation. Apply with a brush and use a sponge to blend. Don't apply to the neck – stop just under the jaw line.

Blush

Blush could be your secret weapon in looking well when you aren't feeling your best. It can give you back your rosy glow. Choose a colour that is warmer than your foundation but not strikingly different. You want the blush to blend, not to stand out.

Apply, using a brush, to the apple on each cheek and blend along the cheek. Make brush strokes in both directions (towards the nose and towards the ears).

Bronzer

Bronzer helps to make you look sun-kissed. It is best applied, lightly, to the areas of the face that naturally catch the sun (the forehead, cheeks, nose and chin).

Don't go too dark. You might be pale underneath but overcompensating with dark colours won't look natural. Stick with one shade darker than your natural colour.

As with blush and foundation, use a brush to apply and a sponge to blend.

Eyeshadow

You may lack the confidence to enhance your eyes, fearing that it will draw attention to your brow and lash areas. The opposite is true: concentrate on your eyes and be brave with your eyeshadow.

Make-up artist Fiona Brunt suggests her favourite look:

'This is easy to achieve and suits everyone. Experiment – be bold or more subtle depending on the occasion.'

- Take an eyeliner powder and apply using a damp brush.
- Wiggle it along your top lashes/lash line. Choose a brown if you want to be more subtle, or black is great if you are feeling a bit bolder. Don't worry about getting a perfect line – just make sure you get it right down to your lash line.
- Place your ring finger just under your brow and gently pull your eyelid upwards so you can see just under your lashes. Fill in any skin you see underneath. Create a solid line to give an illusion of lashes.
- Take your eyeshadow on an eyeshadow brush and gently smudge the eyeliner line up towards your eye crease (or to

your brow if you are feeling bold). The most intense colour should be near the lash line. Blend upwards, softening the colour as you go.

- Use bronze, browns and golds to keep things classic. These shades will flatter almost everyone. However, if you are feeling more adventurous, go for deep purples, blues and greens.
- Make your eyes stand out by choosing the shade which suits your eye colour.
- Use your eyeliner on the bottom lashes/ lash line. Colour in any skin you can see around the lash line.
- Use the same shadow as the top lid to smudge the eyeliner out slightly, but make sure not to bring it too far down below the eye.
- Add more definition by applying a darker shade of eyeshadow onto the outer third of your lid. Blend the shadows so that you don't see any lines.
- Highlight your eyes and make them 'pop'

by adding silver or white to the inner corners of each eye.

If you don't feel that a bold look is for you, Antonia Rudebeck, a make-up artist who works with clients at Leaders in Oncology Care (LOC) on London's Harley Street, suggests 'nude eyes':

- Apply your foundation to your face and eyelid. Leave the area under the eye until last.
- If you have dark circles beneath or around your eyes, camouflage them by mixing yellow mineral powder colour concealer with some of your foundation powder.
- Use black waterproof eyeliner just underneath the lash line of your top lid, creating a lash illusion.
- Apply a neutral brown-tone liner on the top lash line and blend upwards.
- Cover the eye with a matt neutral cream eyeshadow.
- Blend a matt neutral brown tone in the socket.

- Apply brown eyeliner on the bottom lash line.
- Create your brow as illustrated in the Brush-a-Brow guide.

Lips

Lips are often damaged as a side effect of chemo. Lip condition can be improved by applying a natural lip balm twice a day from the start of chemotherapy.[21,]

Your lip health is more important than lipstick. A good natural lip balm can make your lips feel better.[21] The colour in lipsticks, even natural lipsticks, can be drying and is best avoided if your lips are dry and sore. Applying lipstick over lip balm is a good idea if you really do want some colour. Lip gloss, however, is sticky; many wig wearers prefer not to use a gloss, as wigs are infrequently cleaned and gloss can catch the wig hair.

If you feel that your lips are in good enough condition for lipstick, choose your colour according to the occasion and the rest of your 'look'. If you were bold with your eyes, tone down the lips and go for neutral 'nude' shades. If you are wearing a patterned outfit and a red beany, you have to have red lips!

The last word on make-up should go to Melissa Lakersteen, a make-up artist who has worked on film series such as James Bond, Harry Potter and Tomb Raider:

'The most important thing is to stand back and take a really good look at what the make-up is doing for your appearance. Be sure that it is doing what you want it to do. If it's not going as planned, take it off and start again.

'When I make someone up I often take away some of the make-up to adjust the look. Even the professionals don't get it right first time. Don't be afraid to rub some away if it's not doing what you expected it to do.'

A Note About Hygiene

Your immunity is low and you are more prone to infection than usual. Your make-up brushes, sponges and cosmetics can harbour bacteria.

Make sure you clean your brushes and sponges: if possible, boil them. Boiling your brushes and sponges will shorten their life but it is worth it.

When cleaning your brushes with boiling water, don't hold them upright, otherwise the water will reach the dense part of the brush. This area won't dry and the damp bristles will encourage the growth of bacteria.

Always use make-up that is within its recommended period after opening. (Have a look at Appendix 8 if labels are a mystery to you.)

Natural mineral make-up is less able to harbour bacteria. I suggest that you use such a range for the duration of your treatment.

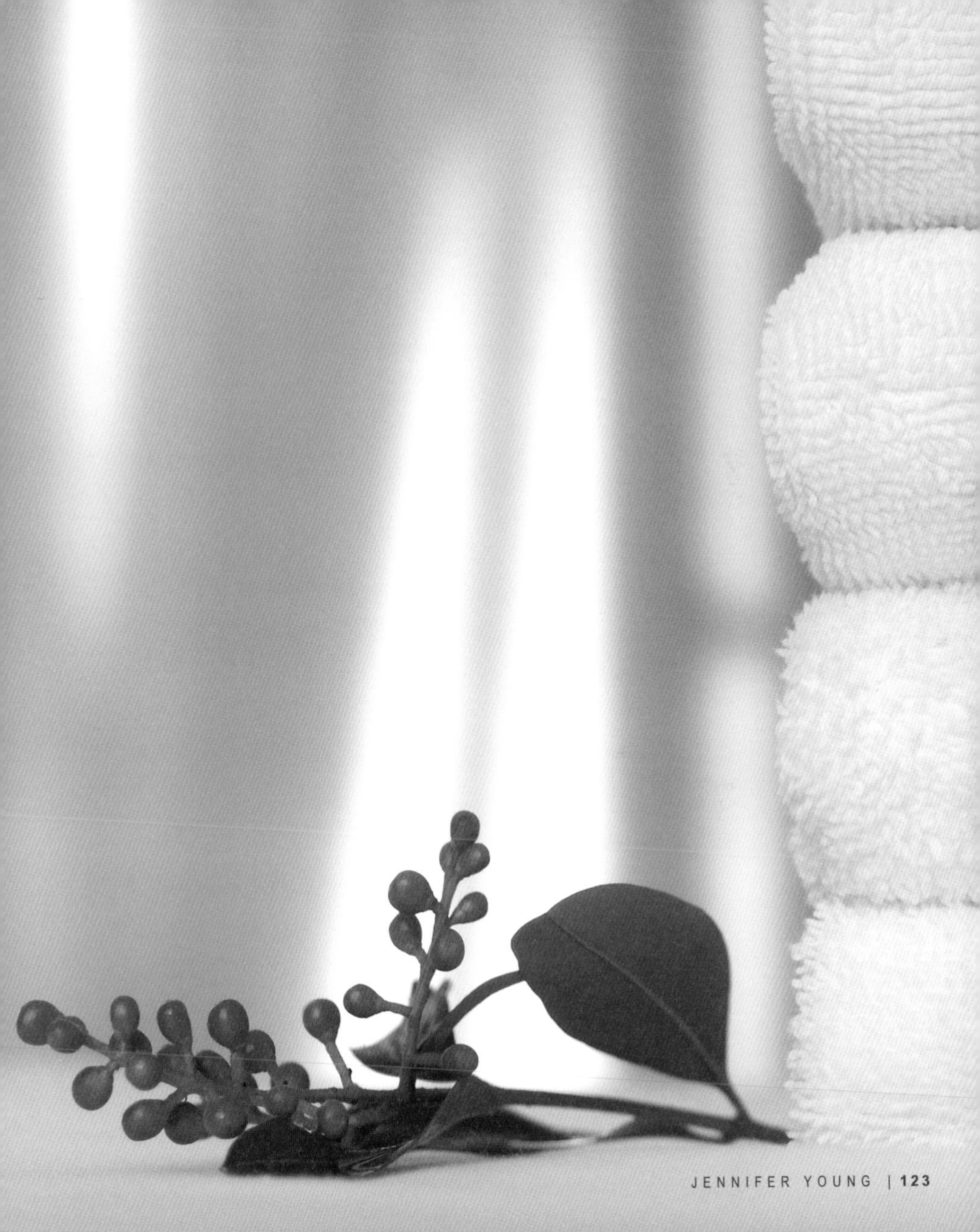

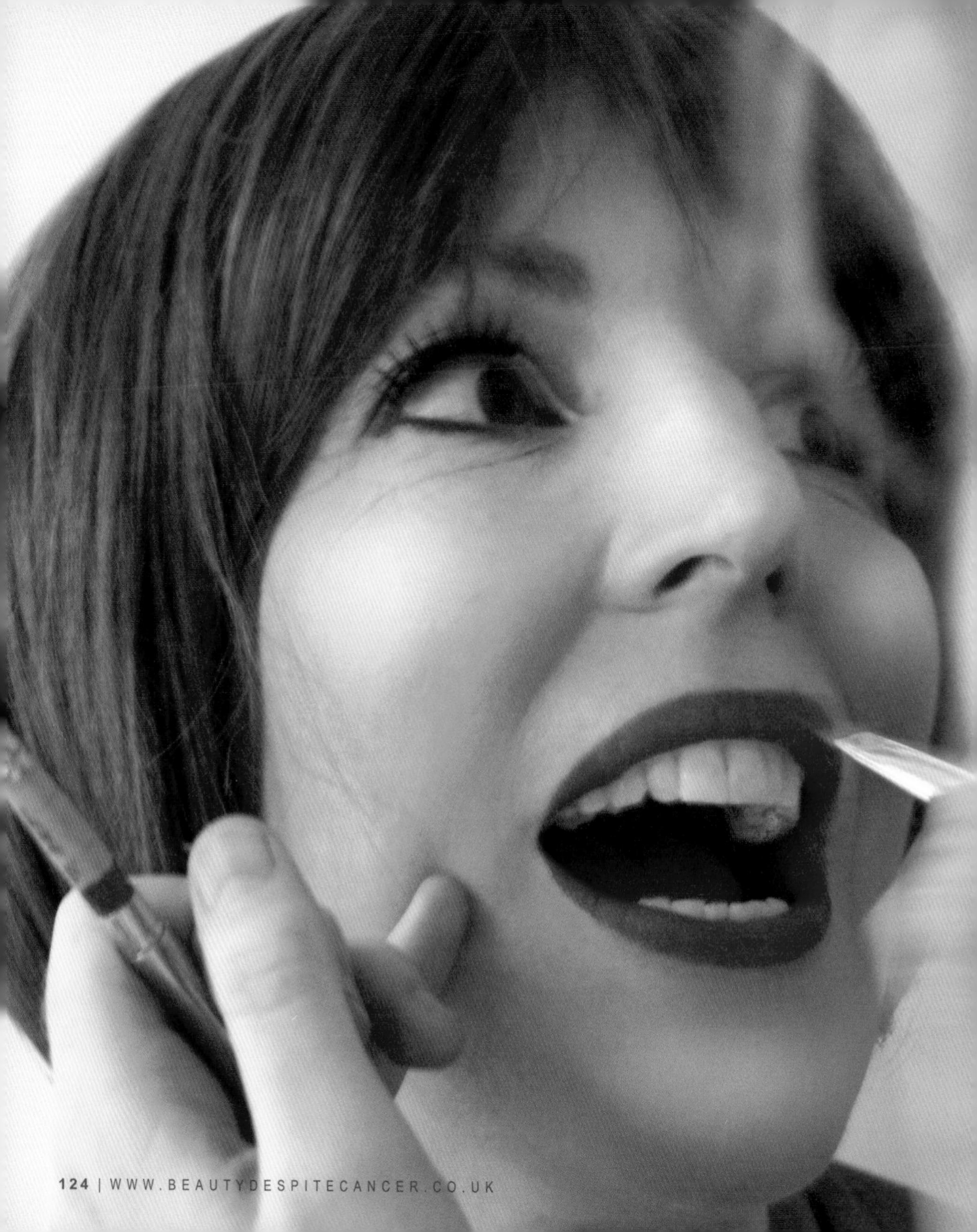

Mouth

Oral and Dental Health

A diagnosis closely followed by a trip to the dentist might not seem like you are doing yourself any favours, but you will be glad that you went.

Dr Harris, a cosmetic dental specialist who works with cancer patients, suggests that a visit as soon as possible after diagnosis is your best option:

'Before any medical treatment it's advisable to be as fit and healthy as possible, and that includes your teeth. Understandably, lots of people, forget about dental treatment when they receive their diagnosis.

'Once treatment has started in earnest it may be difficult to find time to visit the dentist. Good dental habits reduce the chances of future dental problems. It makes sense to visit your dentist in order to take advantage of the latest preventive techniques, before you begin treatment.

'Some large metal fillings can interfere with radiotherapy and may need replacing before

radiation treatment begins. Equally, radiotherapy can impact upon bone healing even when treatment is over. This affects healing after extractions. It makes good sense to have any damaged teeth repaired in advance. Really bad teeth should be extracted at least two weeks before treatment starts.'

Even if you aren't having radiotherapy, a trip to the dentist is a good idea. There can be significant changes in the mouth as a result of treatment. Dr Harris adds:

'Most chemotherapy will leave the soft tissues of the mouth fragile and sore, meaning that brushing and cleaning may be uncomfortable. A dry mouth is often a symptom that has a big impact on tooth decay. It makes sense to get your teeth into the best condition possible before your treatment starts.'

Sucking on ice throughout chemotherapy can reduce damage to the mouth.[22] Both Dr Harris and Prof. Thomas agree that ice is better for this purpose than sugary icicles or ice lollies made from fruit juice.

Dr Harris recommends sucking on slivers of

ice, rather than crunching on ice cubes. The force required to crush an ice cube is greater than that required to crack a tooth. Biting the ice might result in a broken tooth and another trip to the dentist.

The great news is that, generally, there is no need to find a new dentist. Your usual dentist is more than capable of helping you throughout your treatment.

It might make sense for you to attend more frequently than your usual six-monthly appointments, as some of the side effects associated with chemotherapy can make regular dental care difficult. General soreness inside the mouth and reduced saliva flow can result in painful fungal infections and increased tooth decay, and crowns and fillings may not last as long.

Your dentist will liaise with your medical team if any significant dental treatment is required and refer you to a specialist should you need one.

Cosmetic Dentistry

Some chemotherapy treatments can result in darker teeth, and it is natural for you to want to get your teeth 'pearly white' once again. As with all dental treatments, the main issue is whether you feel strong enough to undergo tooth whitening during treatment or whether you wish to wait till your treatment is completed. Dr Harris tells me that tooth whitening is usually well tolerated.

As long as you are happy and the cancer specialists agree that treatment is possible, then any dental treatment can be carried out.

With correct preventive dental care, most potential problems can be overcome. It is best to get in early, though, so don't delay in making your appointment. It could mean fewer trips to the dentist in the future. If you have any concerns about anything, consult with your dentist and your medical team. Appendix 9 contains further information on good dental hygiene.

'You may feel that cosmetic dental treatment is "non-essential", but a lovely smile can lift spirits in much the same way as a wig can help you to feel better about your hair loss.'

Dr Ken Harris, Riveredge Cosmetic Dentistry, Sunderland.

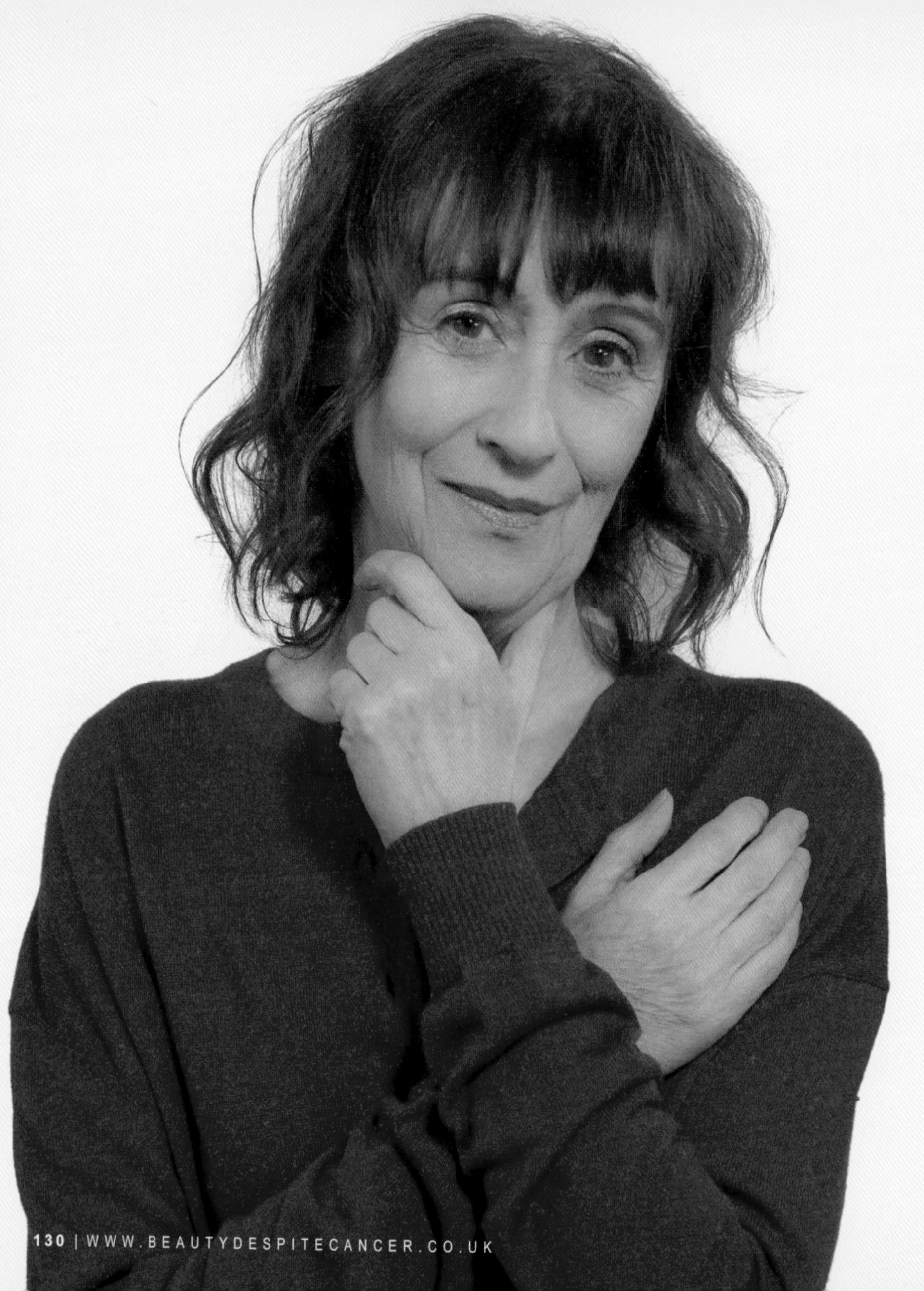

BODY

Body, Hands and Feet

Just as the skin on your face can change, the skin on your body can change too. It may become itchy and sore. Some people experience a greater severity of change than others. As with the face and the scalp, it is important to moisturise the skin.

Nuala Close, the matron of the London Clinic on Devonshire Place, London, has some advice for those with more severe skin reactions. She suggests that patients for whom a bath is painful use a barrier cream to cover their body before they get into the bath. In this way a bath can be enjoyed without discomfort. The matron is keen to stress that one must be careful when trying to bathe while covered in barrier cream – bath time could get a bit slippery and messy. We are also reminded that creams should not be used on broken or irradiated skin.

Hands and Feet

Intense moisturising[14,23] as well as cooling[24] can help sore and blistered skin on the hands and feet.

It is worth revisiting the subject of cooling, which has already been covered in Chapter 1 with regard to hair loss. The same type of treatment can prevent damage to nails and skin on the hands and feet.[24] Cooling gloves and slippers are available in some hospitals. However, there are some conditions for which they are not appropriate, and some medical teams do not recommend them at all.

Again, they are expensive, they require additional time from the nursing or care staff and they are uncomfortable. There is only one choice of gloves and slippers (they look like hand- or foot-shaped cooling packs). If your medical team do recommend gloves and slippers, and you can tolerate them, your hand, foot and nail condition will be improved compared with that of people who do not use them.[24]

If the skin on your hands and feet becomes dry, blistered or sore, ask your medical team if you can apply a thick layer of a soothing natural balm. Cover with cotton gloves or socks before bed and sleep with the hands and feet covered. Make sure you patch test before applying a thick layer.

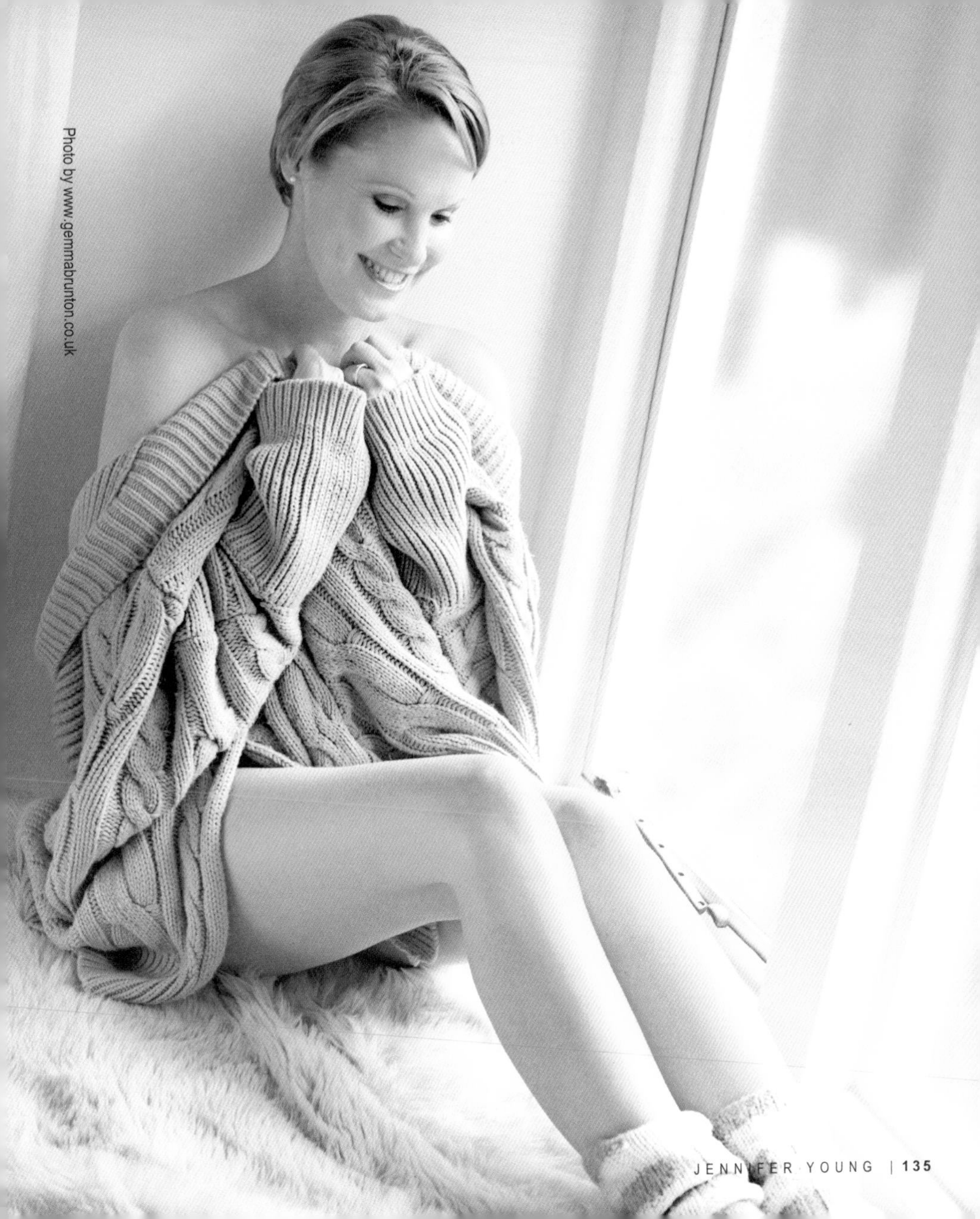
Photo by www.gemmabrunton.co.uk

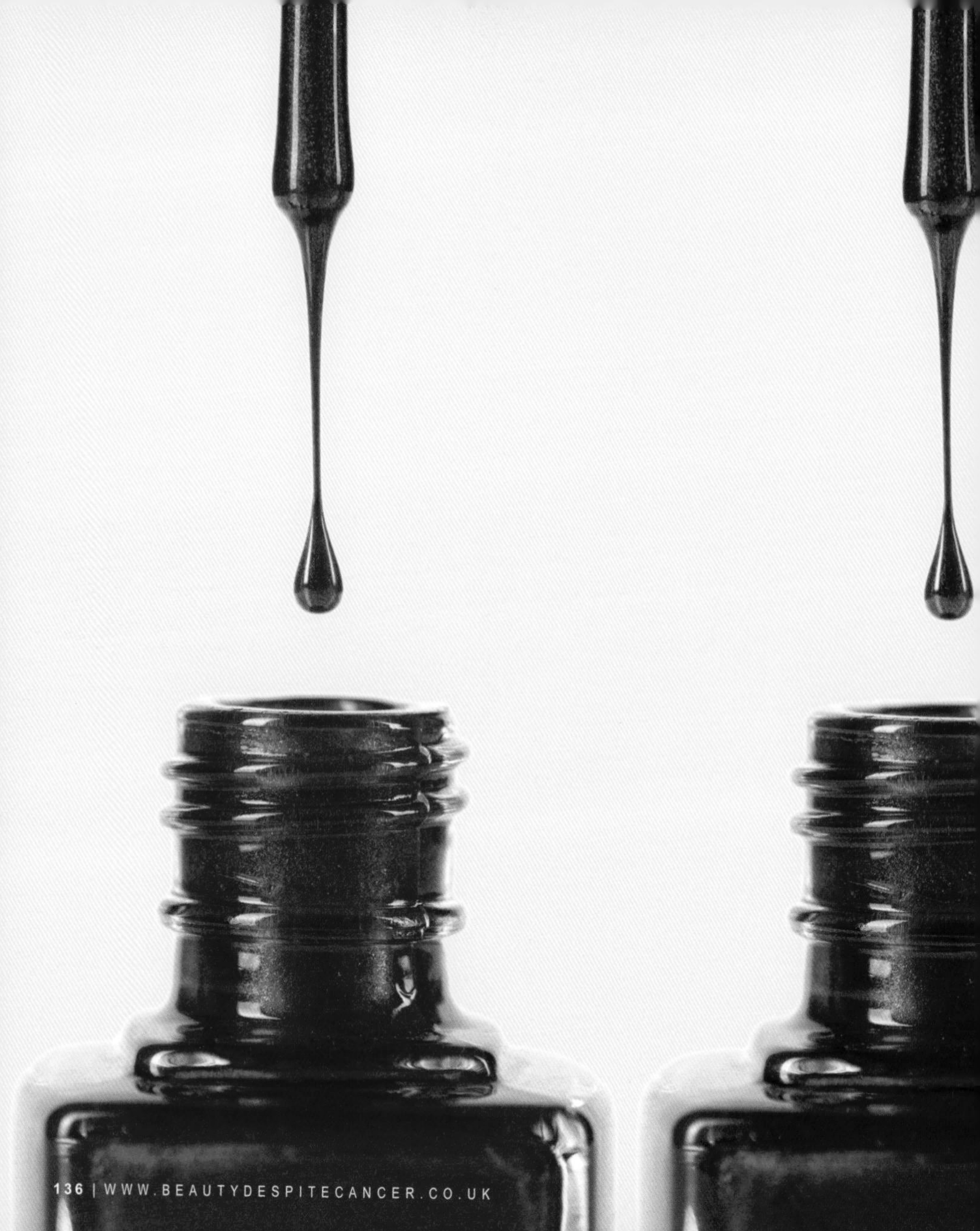

Nails

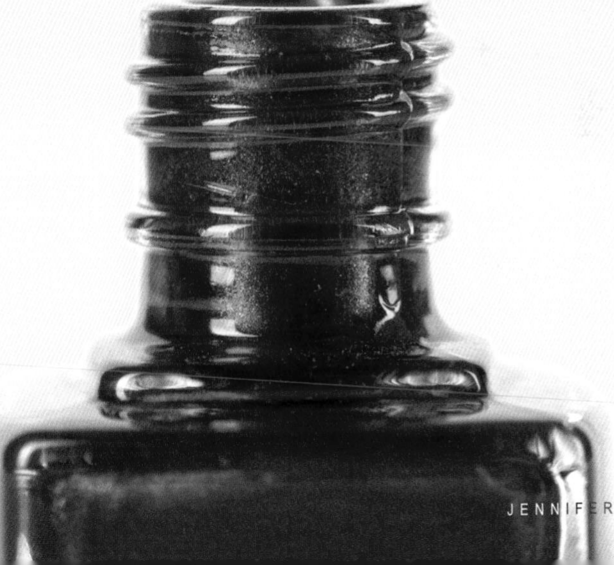

Nails

You are in a minority if you don't have anything done to your nails. In 2013, an estimated 14.5 million people used nail varnish in the UK alone, with an estimated 2.1 million of us being classed as heavy nail varnish and care product users.[25]

Nail salons in the USA generated approximately $8.54 billion in 2014.[26] Nails are big business – most of us love having our nails done.

It is possible that chemotherapy will damage your nails, but don't worry – there are steps that you and your medical team can take to reduce[24] or camouflage[27] damage if it does occur.

If you don't normally apply anything to your nails, you may find that using nail varnish as you go through treatment helps you to disguise some of its side effects. Your nails will return to normal after treatment. You will soon be able to admire your beautiful natural look again. In the meantime, you may prefer to use a coloured nail varnish.

As with hair, plan ahead to reduce and possibly prevent damage.

Cooling

Cooling gloves and slippers can help to reduce nail (and nerve) damage as well as damage to the skin on the hands and feet.[24] Cooling is not appropriate in all circumstances and you will need the consent and support of your medical team in order to use cooling gloves and slippers.

Nail Care

I know I keep mentioning it, but your immunity is low. Your nail care needs to reflect this changed immunity as you go through treatment. Your nails will still look fabulous – worry not.

The wonderful Helen and Alison from Pink Nails run nail care workshops at New Cross Hospital in Wolverhampton. They are both very experienced nail technicians who came to nails from professional backgrounds after Alison's brush with cancer, many years ago. They are the experts in nail care during treatment. This is their advice:

- Use gauze and nail varnish remover to get rid of any existing nail varnish.
- Protect your cuticles by covering the 'hoof' end of an orange stick with cotton wool. Use the stick to gently push back your cuticles – don't cut your cuticles.
- Shape your nails using a glass nail file. Glass nail files will take away length and seal the end of the nail at the same time. Never use a metal file, as these damage your already fragile nails.
- File your nail by placing the glass nail file underneath the nail and 'wiggling'. It is most efficient to file in long strokes from the edge of the nail towards the middle.
- Apply a nail oil.
- Clean the nail again using gauze. Don't use cotton wool, as it can leave hairs on the nails.

- When you are sure the nails are clean, apply a base coat – your nail varnish will last longer if you use a base coat.
- Choose your nail varnish colour. Apply the product sparingly. Make sure there are no 'blobs' on the brush by wiping it against the neck of the bottle until only a small amount of nail varnish remains.
- Place the brush in the centre of the nail and push the colour towards the cuticles.
- Don't try to achieve the perfect coat. Any imperfections will be evened out by the second coat – have faith.
- Apply a second coat of nail colour.
- Apply a top coat to protect the nails and seal at the ends (underneath the top of the nail – the free edge).
- Leave your nails to dry and enjoy.

Nail Oil

Applying nail oil three times a day from the beginning of chemotherapy can reduce the nail-related side effects of the treatment.[27] I find that the oil prolongs the life of a manicure as well.

Acrylic Nails and Gel Nails

It is best to avoid both acrylic nails and gel manicure when you are in treatment. You need to be mindful of your reduced immunity: because these nail types remain on the nail for far longer than nail varnish, they can harbour bacteria that your immune system may struggle to fight.[14]

Salon Nails

Many of us prefer to have our nails done by a professional. Your medical team may advise against a professional manicure or pedicure during treatment, as they are concerned about you picking up an infection.

If this is the case, use the Pink Nails guide to help you to do your own nails. It isn't as daunting as you think – I know ladies who practise their nail art while they have chemotherapy.

If you are able to have a professional manicure, choose your nail technician with great care. Your medical team are right to be cautious. Do not, under any circumstances, let your nail technician cut your cuticles or the skin at the side of the nails. Discuss your needs with them and do not let them touch your nails if you are not confident that they can accommodate your requirements as you go through treatment.

> *'What can I do to help my sister-in-law? She has her nails done every week. She is so proud of her nails. I can't imagine her not having perfect nails.'*
>
> Caller to the Beauty Despite Cancer Appearance Advice Line

A Troubleshooting Guide for Nails Changed by Chemotherapy

CONCERN	ACTION
Fragile nails	Keep nails short. Use nail varnish and nail oil.
Dry nails	Use nail oil.
Flaking nails	Keep nails short. Use nail varnish and nail oil.
Discoloured nail beds	Use a dark nail varnish to camouflage discolouration.
Ridged nails	Use nail oil and a dark, glittery nail varnish to camouflage ridges.

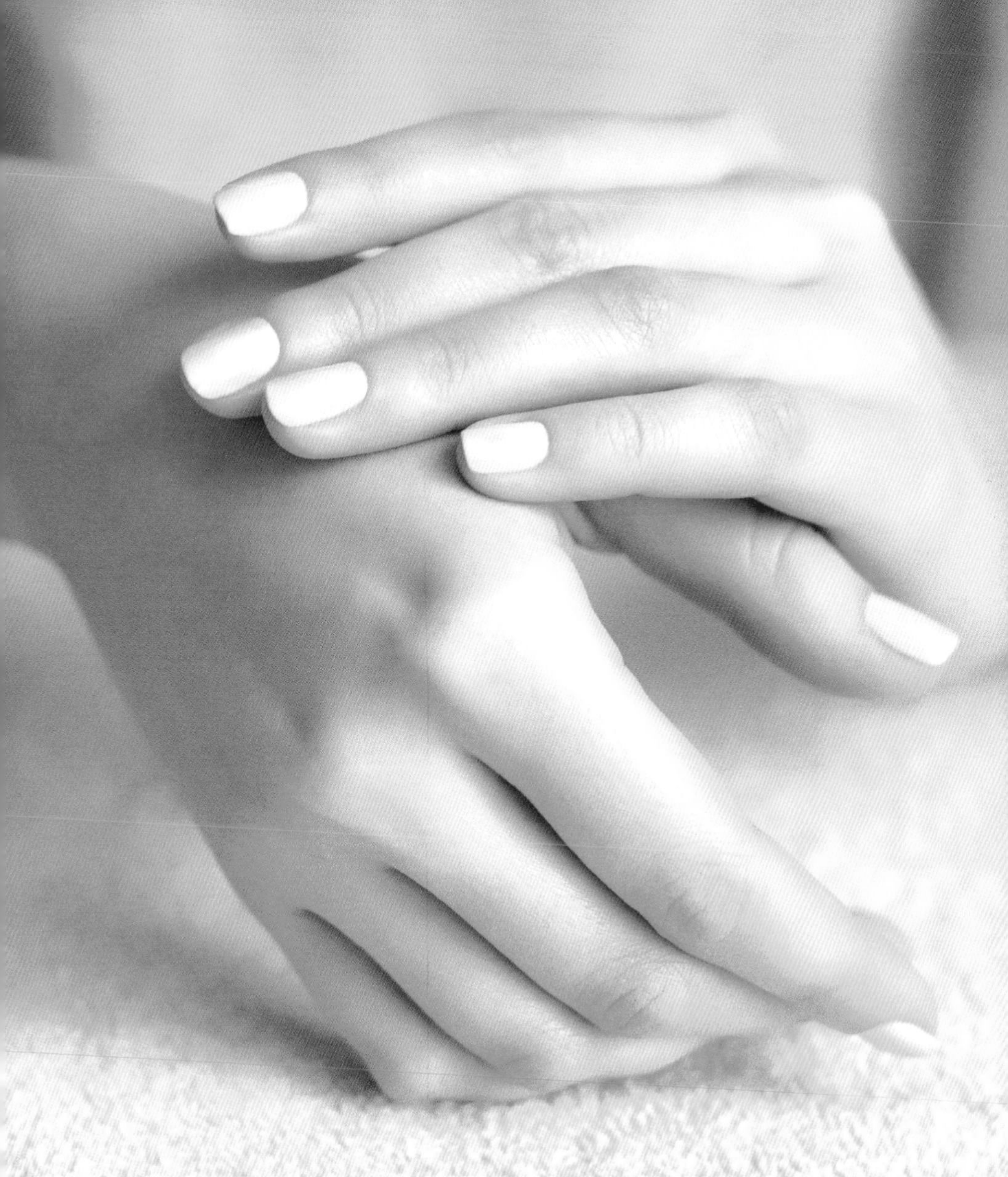

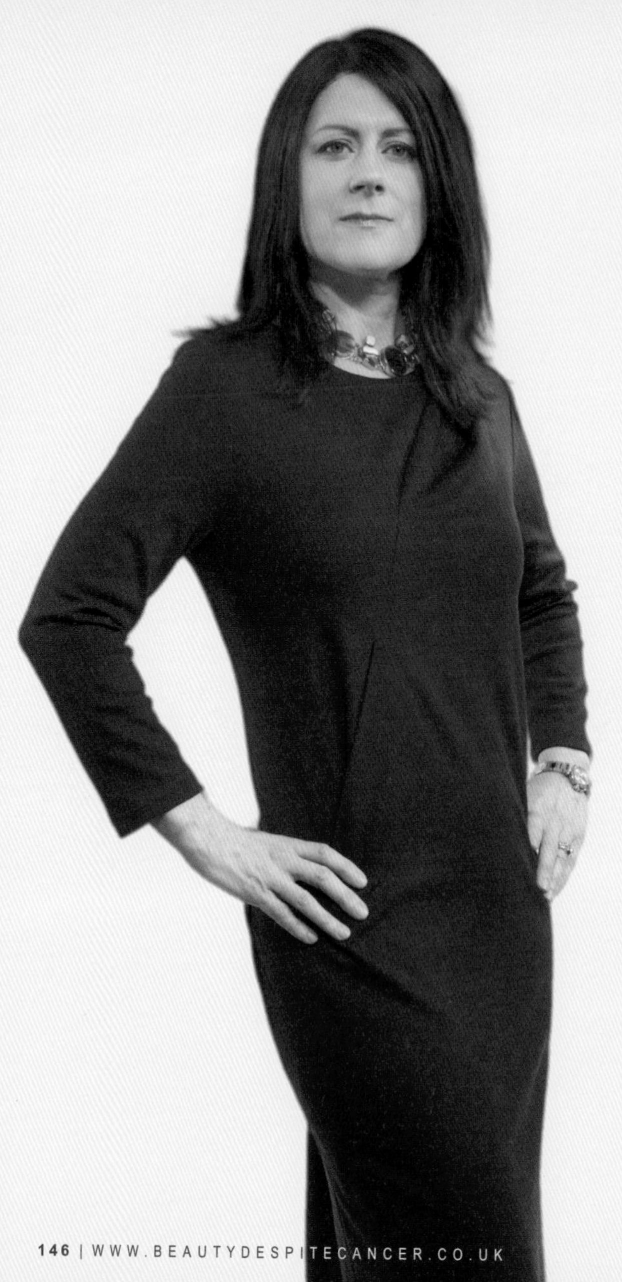

Your Look

How to Dress

I hope I am not alone in finding 'style' at best a mystery, and at worst an ordeal. I am no fan of shopping for clothes and I am happiest in my (very comfortable) gym kit.

When I visit groups of patients, many are exquisitely dressed. Almost all tell me that they feel the need to make more of an effort throughout treatment, as they are facing greater hurdles.

How does one style oneself? Clearly I am not the woman to give that advice. Luckily, I know some ladies who can help, some of whom have shared your experiences.

I realise that my favourite piece of advice, coming from Kaz Molloy, is less relevant anatomically to those who have been through surgery for breast cancer, but I think it is good advice, suited to almost all circumstances.

> *'Wear big, comfortable knickers.'*
>
> Kaz Molloy

Surgery and Body Changes

Surgery has both short-term and long-term effects. In the short term you are likely to be uncomfortable and could have limited mobility.

Anikka Burton had surgery at quite short notice. She remembers not only having to get used to the fact that she was 'ill', but also having to scour the streets looking for pyjamas with a buttoned top. Buttoned pyjamas were recommended by her hospital, as she would be unable to lift her arms for a while after surgery.

Ask your medical team about any predicted limited mobility, as well as for suggestions for nightwear that will accommodate those limitations.

You will want to dress for comfort after surgery – loose waists and baggy tops. Many women find that they are very hot after surgery, so keep this in mind when packing for hospital.

There are many types of cancer and just as many treatment options. Concerns relating to body image tend to be associated with surgery type. This chapter deals mainly, but by no means exclusively, with the body changes necessitated by surgery for breast cancer.

Breast Surgery

Breast surgery has the potential to change body shape. Some women who have had a mastectomy or lumpectomy feel that they are no longer symmetrical.

Scarring may prevent some women from wearing the low-cut tops that they used to enjoy. Because of scars from ports, some cancer patients may not feel comfortable in tops with lower necklines.

Weight Gain or Weight Loss

Weight can be influenced by treatment – some patients find it difficult to eat and so lose weight. Some types of surgery make eating and digestion difficult.

In contrast, other treatment regimes involve steroids and patients can put on weight. A new wardrobe and a new approach to selecting clothes may be necessary.

'A friend looked me up and down very critically and said: "Oh, I always thought cancer was meant to make you lose weight." Luckily I've got a sense of humour.'

Yvonne Newbold, London

Colour and Complexion

The camouflaging of changed colour and complexion has been covered in Chapter 2.

You can use make-up to make you look well, but you will look even better if you use style to your advantage.

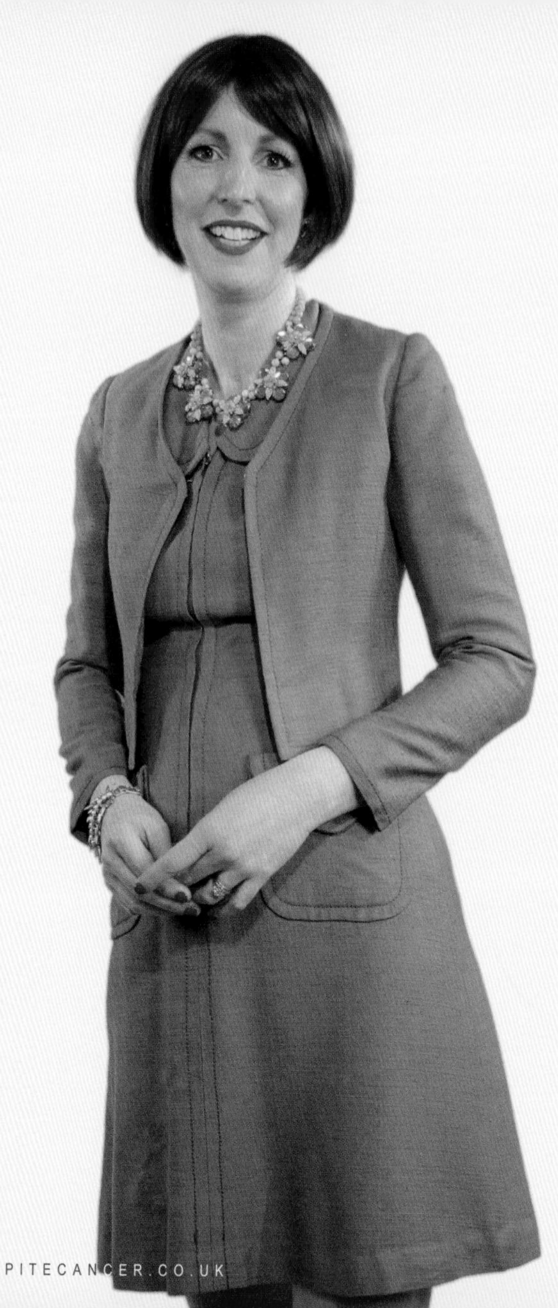

Style

Style

According to Melissa Lackersteen of Make Up Matters, the first basic rule of style is to know your colours. If, like me, you have no idea of your colours, the best way to discover them is to visit a style consultant. However, you can do it yourself if you prefer – here's how…

Go to a shop and choose clothes of very different colours (no patterns yet). Place them under your face and see which suits you best. For the moment, put aside your feelings about wearing the colours. Notice how well you look when you have different colours beneath your chin and make a note of those which make you glow. There will be a big difference in how you look in different colours. Spend some time learning about what suits you.

When you have your colours sorted, it's time to discover which styles suit your new body shape. Dress for the body you have, not the body you want or the body that you used to have. There is every chance that you will achieve the body shape you want but, for now, work with what you have.

Entire books have been devoted to matching style to body shape. I asked Melissa to help us out with some basic rules:

- Decide which areas you want to accentuate and which you want to draw attention away from. If you are concerned about being asymmetrical in the chest area, divert attention away from that area.
- An asymmetrical style will camouflage any unevenness in the body. Asymmetry may be found in a hemline, in detail on a top, or in a design.
- Draw the eye away from areas that you would prefer not to emphasise, by wearing big jewellery or a short skirt, or by utilising a design detail such as pockets.
- If you have a small waist, choose something to emphasise it, so taking attention away from your chest. Long legs can be accentuated, as can curves.

I appreciate that it can take a lot of time and effort to discover your style. Women who have invested that time tell me that it is time well spent and that it saves them a fortune.

'Everyone has colours that help them to look their best. As soon as you discover them, life is easier. If facial colour and complexion change, the colours that suit you best could also change. Bear this in mind if you knew your colours prior to treatment.'

Melissa Lackersteen, style consultant, Make Up Matters

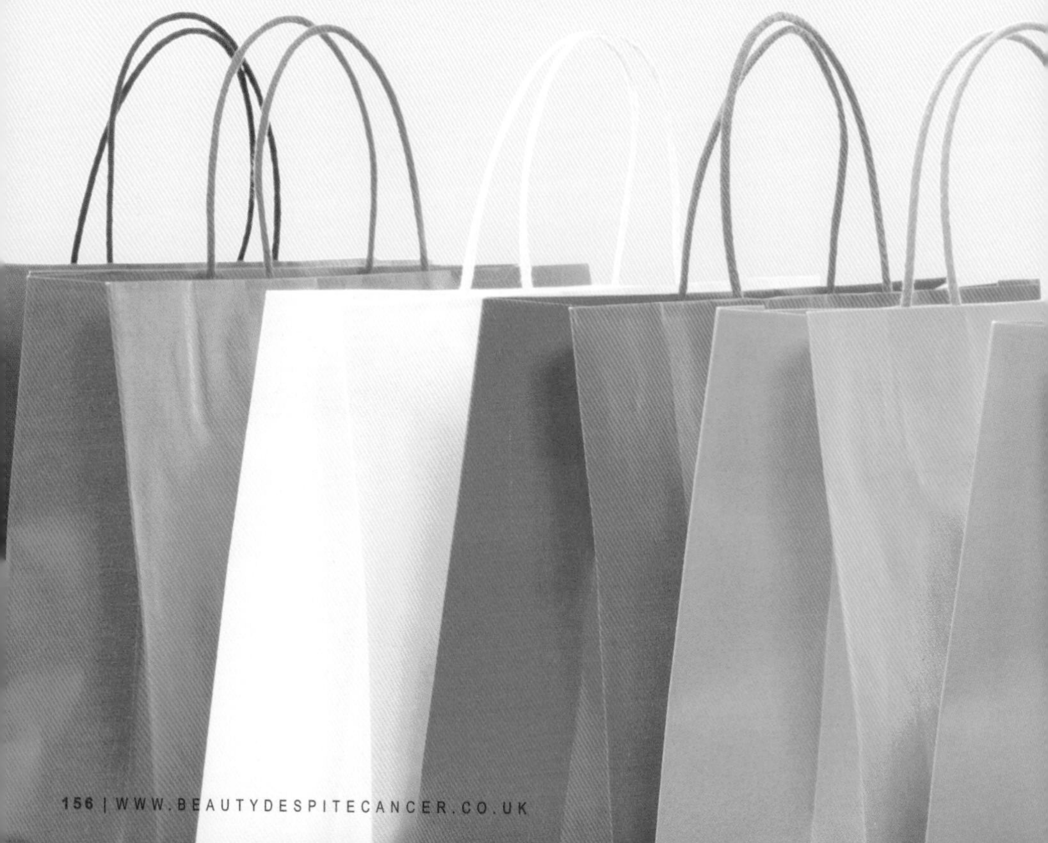

'Our bra-fitting events are great fun. A group of ladies join us when the boutique has closed for the evening. We have nibbles and fizz and offer fittings (in the private fitting rooms).

'We thought that breast cancer patients would prefer not to have a special event, but we have found that they appreciate being with people who have had similar experiences. Everyone has some supportive and useful advice. It's never just about bras.'

Paula and Lisa, Embrace, Worcester

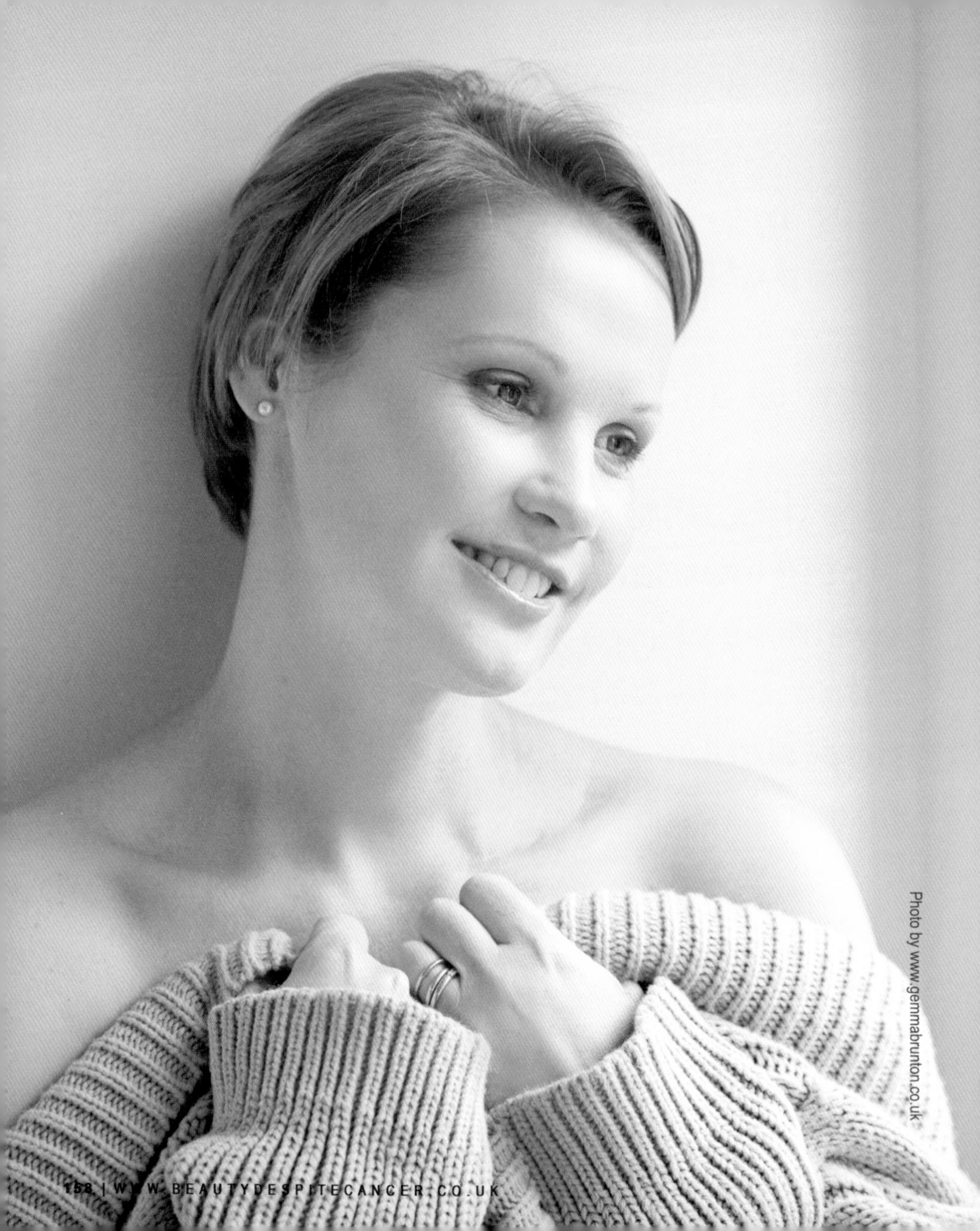
Photo by www.gemmabrunton.co.uk

Lingerie

Lingerie

What do you mean that you need a bit more advice than Kaz Molloy's suggestion to 'wear big knickers'?

Lingerie, a pleasure in good times, can become overwhelming in really bad times. You need specialist help in deciding on the best lingerie for you, particularly if you have had breast surgery.

Anita, a German company, is the biggest supplier of post-operative and mastectomy lingerie to the UK. They provide training to their stockists and very kindly invited to me to one of their training days. Their advice for those living with and beyond breast cancer is as follows.

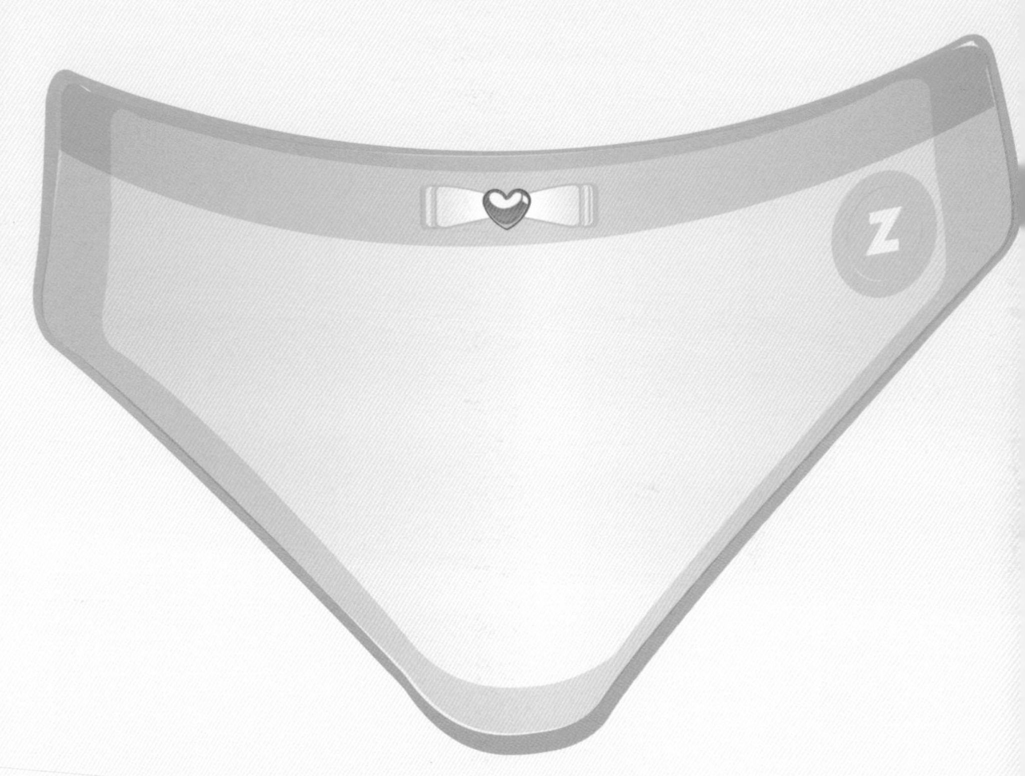
Z

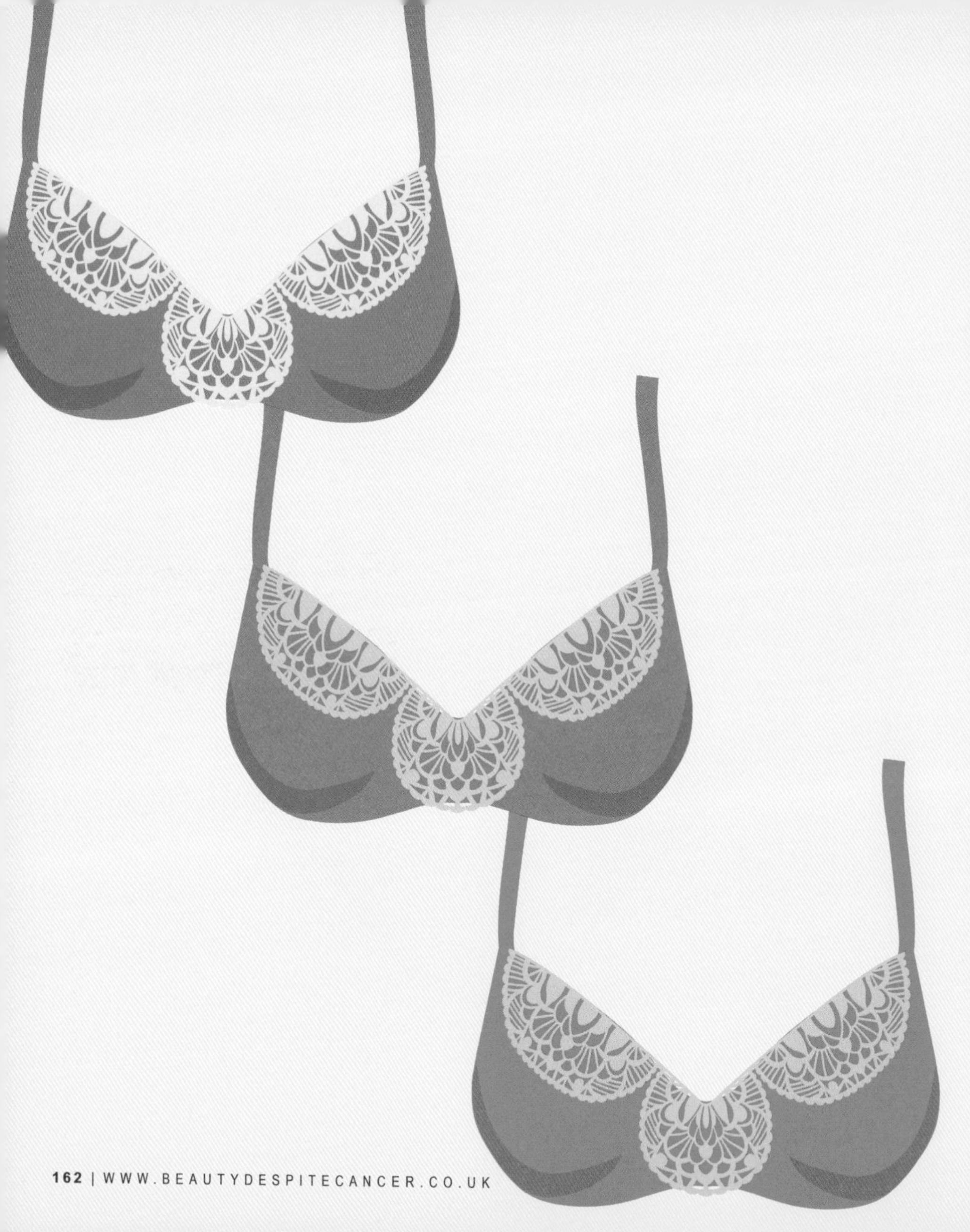

Bras

Post-operative Bras

There is a selection of bras that will help keep you comfortable and well supported after surgery. Some of these post-operative bras are designed specifically for where reconstruction has taken place and feature compression for wound healing; others have seam-free interiors and soft touch for those undergoing radiotherapy. A third type of bra has soft front fastening and is pocketed. The pockets hold a soft breast form and help support the remaining breast during the healing process. Approximately three months after surgery, the move to pocketed bras for all occasions can be made.

The consultation process is key when recommending a pocketed bra for a post-surgery customer. After the scarring has healed, there are many products that would not be comfortable; some could even create complications.

Most surgeons recommend that a non-wired bra should be worn. Bras without an underwire are more comfortable and reduce the risk of future complications.

However, post-surgery bras are not simply non-wired bras with a pocket – there is much more to consider, not least the risk of lymphoedema (a fluid retention that causes a swelling to the arm).

The risk of lymphoedema is higher in ladies who have had lymph nodes removed as part of their surgery. Where this is the case, not only should the bra be non-wired but it should also be free of any side stiffeners sewn into the underarm area. Ideally the bra should be seam free or have a covered seam in the underarm area.

The most important things to look for in a post-surgery bra are the following:

- Soft fabric
- Deeper than average underarm bands (for comfort over scar tissue)
- Deeper centre cores (for separation of the breast/breast form)
- Higher décolleté, for coverage and containment of the breast form and to prevent it from moving around

- A defined underband to anchor the bra and give comfort without too much pressure
- Broad/padded straps for comfort and prevention of lymphoedema.

Sue Pringle has been through treatment for cancer twice: she has had two lumpectomies, a mastectomy, a reconstruction and two menopauses. Sue is on a mission to create a better bra. Her quest stems from her own experiences, conversations and research. Sue found that bra buying escalates soon after surgery:

'You will probably find that you need to buy more bras than usual in the period immediately following your surgery. Your breast size may continue to fluctuate for up to a year, depending on your subsequent treatment. The swelling caused by lumpectomy surgery can last for up to three months, and radiotherapy can cause fluctuations in breast size for a year or so. It's also worth considering possible weight gain.'

Mastectomy Bras

A mastectomy bra is different from a post-surgery bra. It looks like any other bra but contains cup linings or pockets to contain a breast prosthesis (an artificial breast form that replaces the shape of all or part of the breast that has been removed).[28]

Sue Pringle tells us more about prostheses:

'A high proportion of women in the UK elect for what is referred to as "breast conserving surgery" or lumpectomy. The breast(s) are reduced in size and shape. There are lots of ways to recreate a more even-looking contour and shape by combining a well-fitting bra with a prosthesis.

'Most NHS breast clinics offer a free prosthesis-fitting service, usually run by a specially trained member of the nursing team. The timing of the fitting varies between health authorities. This can make a difference to the shape you achieve and the bra that will work best for you. Ask about the service when you make your clinic visit after surgery. I wasn't told and made do with uneven-looking breasts when

'Prepare yourself for more frequent replacement of your bras as your needs change.'

Sue Pringle

I needn't have.

'There is a wide range of shapes, sizes and skin tones available, so it's relatively easy to find a prosthesis that's right for you. Most are worn by inserting into a pocketed bra. There are also "sticky" prostheses that are worn directly against the chest wall, making it easier to wear a standard bra. A word of caution – they can become quite hot and very sticky during the summer months, but do give you more bra choices.

'"Softie" prostheses are designed to be worn soon after surgery. As their name suggests, they are softer and more comfortable to wear while things settle down; they can also be worn if only a little extra fullness is required. Softies designed for swimming are also available. As an NHS patient, every woman is entitled to one prosthesis (excluding first softies); after that it's more common to pay for one.'

'It's time for another bra when you feel that you aren't as supported as you were. Perhaps your body shape has changed or your bra has stretched.'

German company Anita

Using the right bra after a double mastectomy and reconstruction is crucial to recovery: it will help the healing process by stabilising the breasts and minimising movement. Movement prevents the wound closing up and results in slower healing; this, in turn, can increase the risk of scarring and infection, and the final breast positions may not be level or balanced.

Surgeons and specialists recommend a compression bra. The controlled and directional compression offers the breasts strong support in the areas where it is needed, and yet the bra is soft and comfortable against the skin and the pressure points that remain sensitive after surgery.

Compression bras are generally front fastening to minimise stretching and to allow ease of putting on; they also feature soft, wide and Velcro-adjustable straps for convenience.

Often compression bras come with the option of a 'belt', which is only used in cases where a silicone or saline implant has been used for the reconstruction. If these implants are not held in place with a belt until they have bedded into the breast and stabilised into a permanent position, they will move as the body moves.

Compression bras, more than anything, 'take the strain', allowing the woman to relax in her natural posture and not hold herself in order to protect her wound or to be comfortable.

I am always amazed that women even attempt to choose and fit their own bras. Don't do it! Go to a specialist and be fitted. Specialist retailers will always have more stock than a general high-street store, and the fitters are likely to be more experienced. They will also be able to help you with a breast prosthesis, should it be appropriate. Often it was the circumstances of these specialist retailers themselves having breast cancer and being unable to find suitable bras and good advice that motivated them to start their own businesses.

Sue Pringle recommends that your bra fit be checked every three months immediately after surgery and every six months after that, but more frequently if there is any significant change in weight.

Recognising yourself is about more than the reflection you see in the mirror - you are dealing with a lot of emotions as well. I cannot help you with emotional concerns, as my expertise is in beauty and skincare.

Thankfully, Beauty Despite Cancer is a collaboration of experts. In the next chapter our experts will share their wisdom regarding emotional aspects.

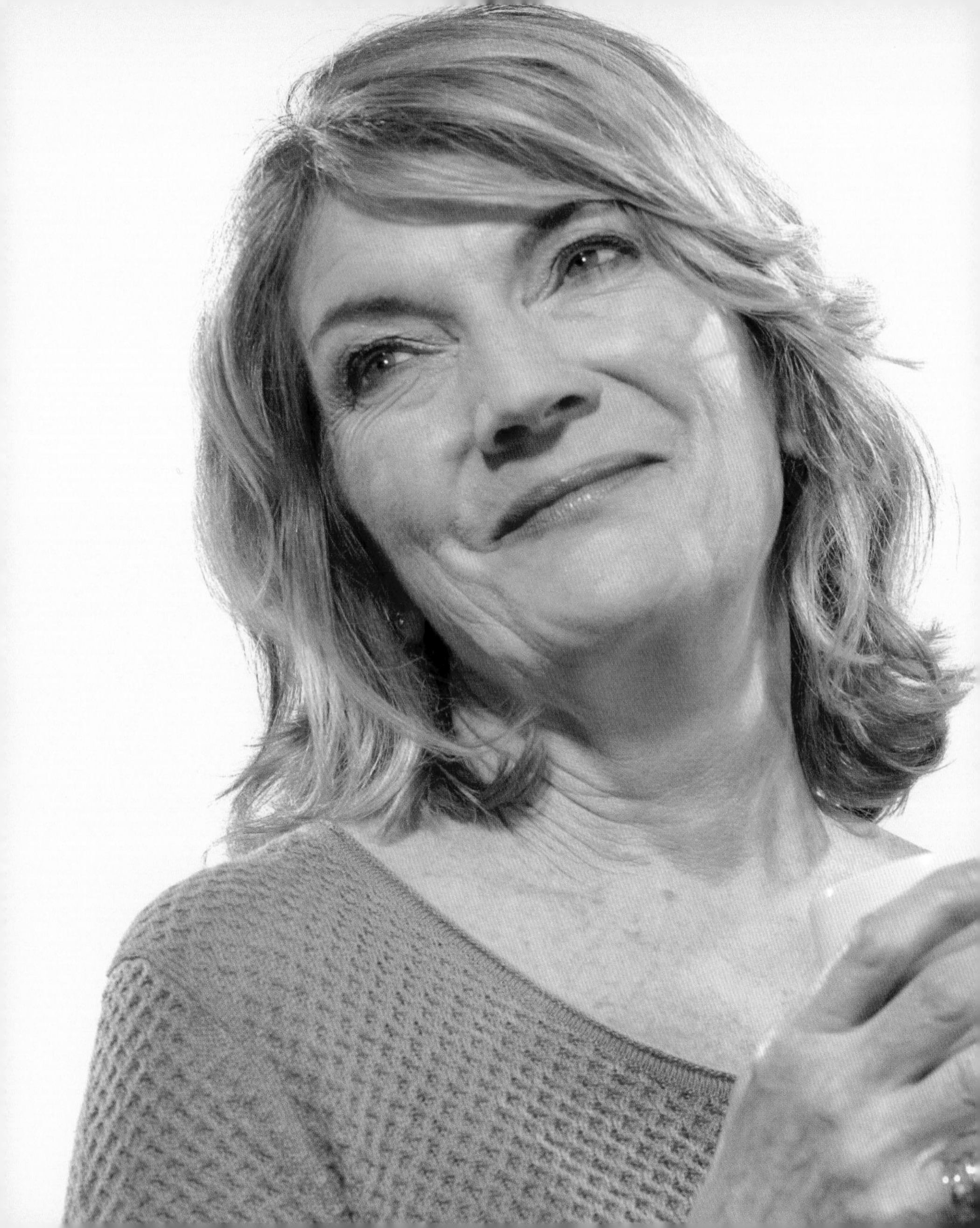

SELF

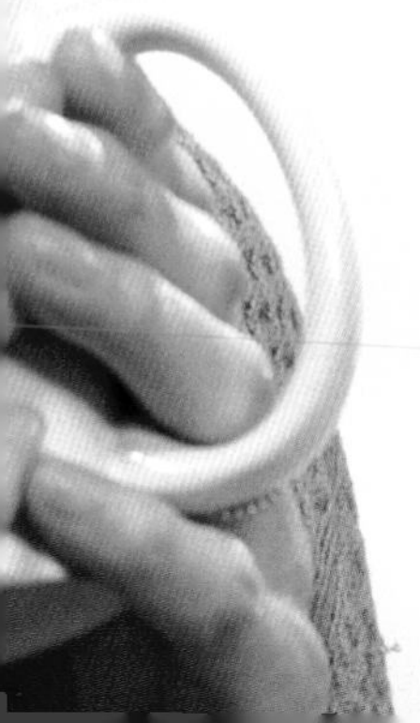

Why Me?

Have you ever asked yourself this? Prof. Robert Thomas of Addenbrooke's Hospital in Cambridge tells me that 'Why me?' is the question most often asked at diagnosis.[2]

Are there any answers to this question? The Rev. David Williams, Lead Chaplain at Alder Hey Children's Hospital, Liverpool, explains that sometimes things happen for no reason:

'Most people look for something to blame – that's a very human thing to do. Our first reaction as humans, when something goes very wrong, or when something doesn't turn out the way we planned, is usually to look for something or someone to blame. We have been hurt and we want to hit out at somebody or something.

'We're not good at accepting that things sometimes just happen. They don't happen to any plan. They don't happen for any reason. They don't happen because of any avoidable action, any defective workmanship or any act of God. Things sometimes just happen.

'And it's the fact that things can sometimes just happen, so randomly, that makes them so difficult to accept, because it reminds us just how powerless we are to really shape our own destinies. Our plans can so easily be knocked off course, leaving us floundering in the wake of some totally random event, and we can do little or nothing about it. We didn't see it coming and we certainly didn't want it. But it's here, and now we just have to deal with it as best we can.

'And that makes us frustrated and that makes us angry. And why shouldn't it?

'When we see people prosper, those who seem to ride roughshod over every value that we hold as decent, then we have a right to feel aggrieved. When we see the fat cats who are happy to profit from the misery inflicted upon others and are enjoying their ill-gotten gains, we have a right to feel cheated. When those who pay no heed to health warnings seem to live life happily to the full while we struggle with health issues despite following all the safety and advisory guidelines, we have a right to feel very resentful.

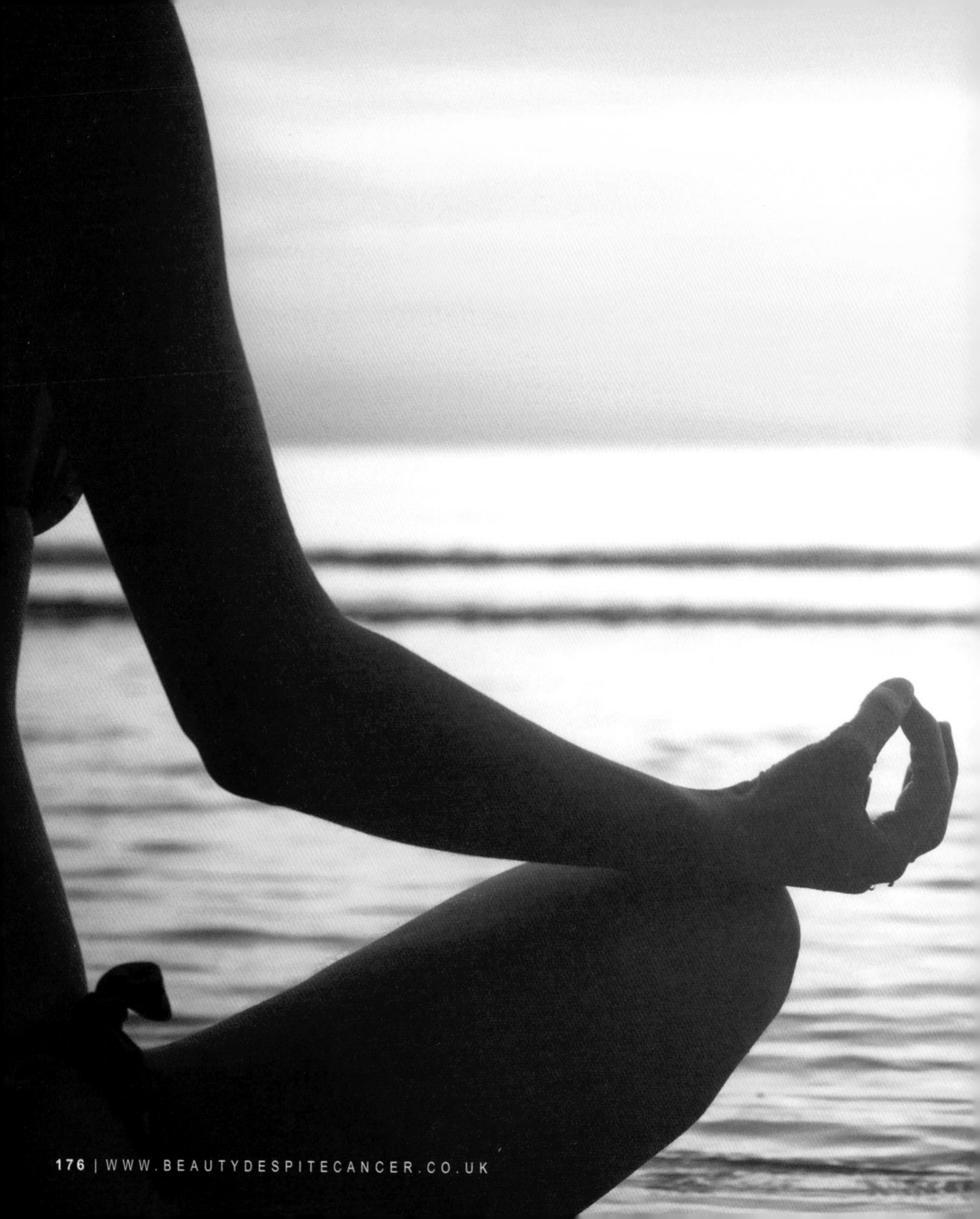

'Life is scary sometimes and,
we don't have all the answers.
But I know that you will find the
strength and the courage that
you need to move on and to face
whatever life throws at you.'

Rev. David Williams

'When cancer finds a way in, then you have every right to be angry and to feel that you have been dealt a really bad hand. And having been dealt such a hand, it's entirely understandable that you feel vulnerable, so fragile, and even resentful. Nor is it surprising in the slightest that you want answers to your hard questions, and you hate the fact that you are simply not in control of your life. It would not be surprising for anyone to react in this way, because we are only human, we are mortal, and when we are faced with these huge questions of life and death, all other matters pale into relative insignificance.

'So we cling as never before to the things that we can control, to the constants in our lives that we can rely on, and for many, one of those constants is our faith in God, or in some force or being that is so much greater than ourselves.'

Helping Patients Through Treatment

Spirituality helps cancer patients through their treatment and is associated with an improved outcome. Patients with what the research terms 'spirituality well-being' are found to have a more positive experience as they go through treatment – they have better coping strategies, feel more positive and are less likely to suffer depression and anxiety.[29-36]

What then if you feel abandoned by your God or the higher forces in which once you had faith? Rev. David Williams gives us his thoughts, based on his experiences as a Christian minister working with the families of very sick children:

'I guess that we are then left with that one great question that you have every right to ask: Why? It is, after all, an entirely valid and relevant question. If God is all-loving and all-powerful, why is this suffering allowed to happen?

'The answer is, I don't know. I don't know why life has to be so unfair sometimes. I don't

know why children get sick, or why some die. I don't know why good people often seem to get the wrong end of the deal, or get dealt bad hands.

'I don't know why, but I do not believe that this is the will of my God or of the other forces in which you believe.

'Why? Because I have to ask myself, if sickness and illness were part of God's plan, why did Jesus heal people? I don't ever see Jesus turning to anybody to say: "It's God's will that you are blind, or that you have leprosy, or that you are lame." Jesus heals them.

'That's why I don't believe that physical illness was ever a part of God's plan in the beginning.

'But I do also know that Jesus never promised us that life would be fair on this earth, and that he never promised that we'd get the hand we wanted. For me, one of the constantly held and repeated illusions of the understanding of Christian teaching is that Jesus somehow promises an easy and carefree life to those who choose to believe in him.

'That's just not true.

'The lives of those who chose and who choose to follow Jesus are often more marked with suffering and hardship on this earth rather than carefree existence. Jesus himself warned that in this world we would have trouble, but that we should not be afraid because he had overcome this world.

'I see that as Jesus saying to us: "I can't get you round these troubles, but I will get you through them."

'And the strength to overcome those troubles is in the belief, or even the knowledge, that God does weep alongside us in the suffering, and that sometimes, despite all appearances, God does care so very, very much.

'Life is scary sometimes and, as I've already said, we don't have all the answers. But I know that you will find the strength and the courage that you need to move on and to face whatever life throws at you.

'And I know that you will not be alone as you put one step in front of the other, because God will be walking alongside you and He will be there to pick you up if you stumble.'

David tells me that the response he hears most often when he offers support is 'But we don't go to church' – a response which to him is entirely irrelevant.

Religion or Faith?

There is a difference between being religious and having a faith or a spiritual belief. Research helps us out.

Religion involves structured worship, theological beliefs, practices and rituals.[37,38] Spirituality may or may not include religion.[37] Spirituality is a search for meaning and purpose. I am no expert but it seems to me, if you ask 'Why me?', you are searching for meaning and purpose. You may find it helpful to recognise your spiritual needs.

Your spiritual needs can be met in any number of ways, organised religion being but one. Research into spirituality and cancer treatment describes spirituality as 'connections to self, others and the world'.[38]

Another study found that patients mentioned spirituality, meaning and purpose in a number of ways, including connecting with family and friends, nature, art, and music. Some created a relationship with God. Others accessed spirituality by enhancing connections in their own lives – with a higher power, people, their work or themselves. These enhanced connections gave a greater meaning and purpose in life, and substantially helped some patients to adjust to their diagnosis and life beyond it.[38]

Something as unlikely as going to a yoga class may help you to connect.

'There are many benefits to yoga –it's a safe and calming place to reconnect with your changing body whilst supported by fantastic people.'

Barbara Gallani, specialist yoga teacher

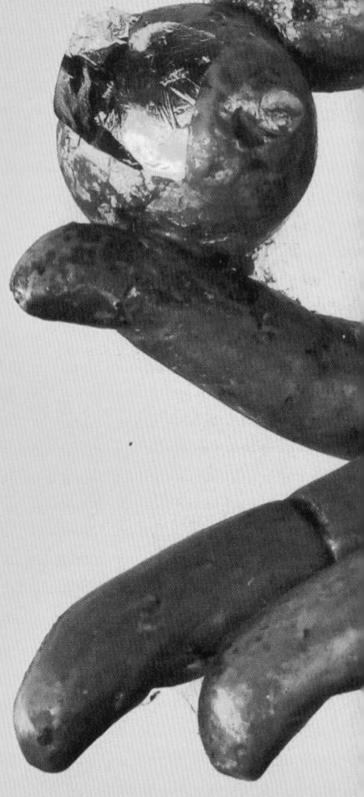

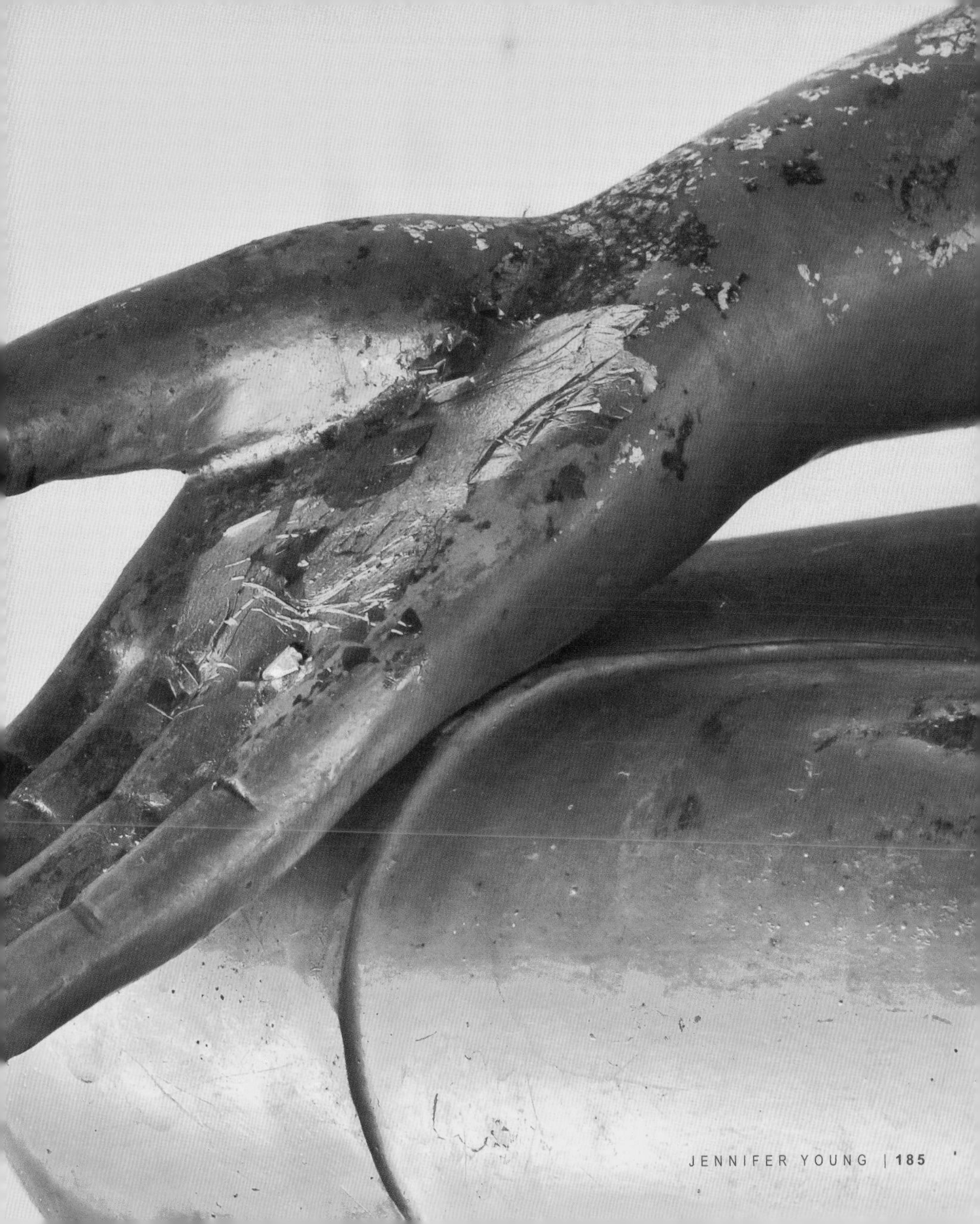

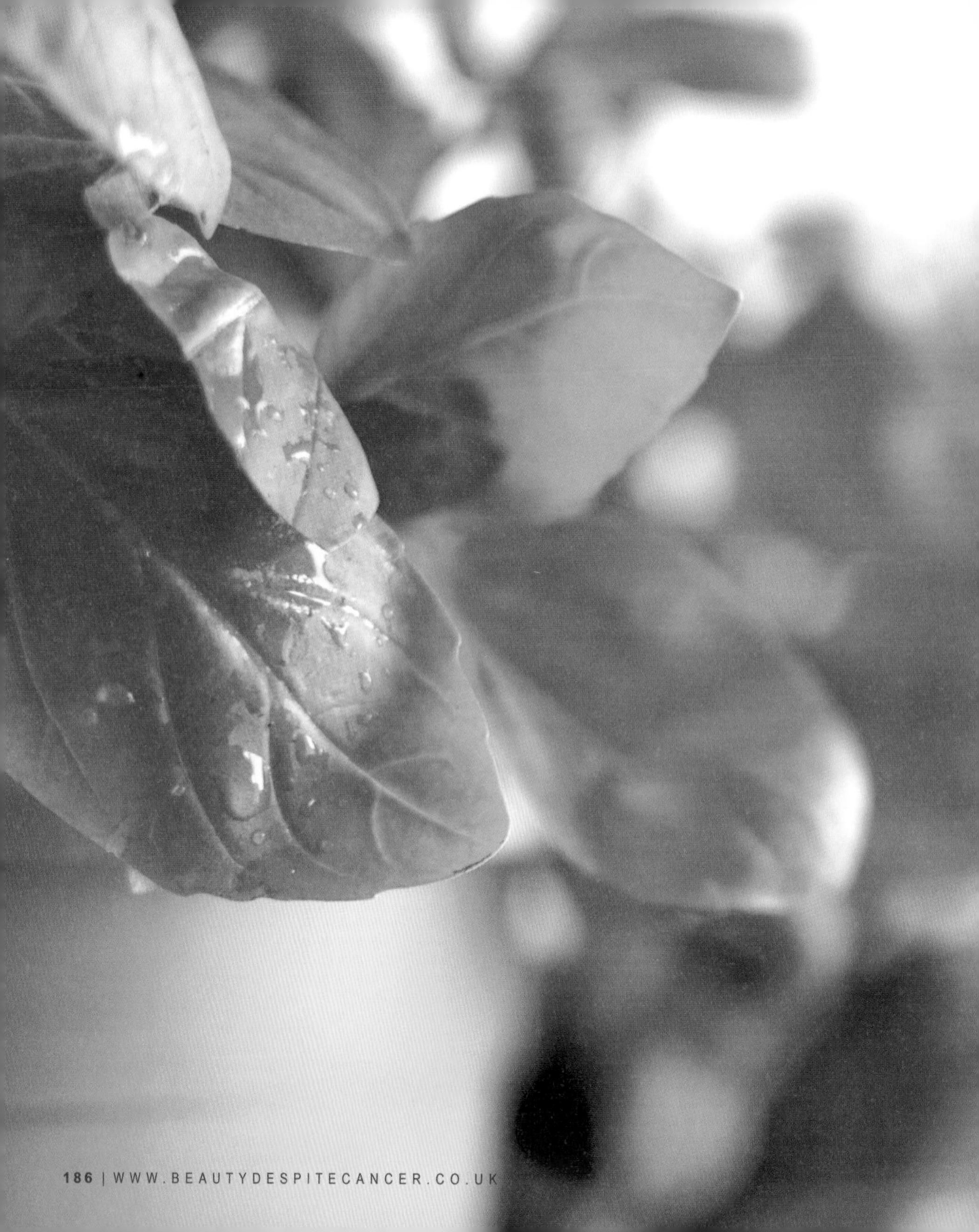

Nutrition

Nutrition

There is a lot of conflicting information about food and nutrition. I find it confusing and I am a qualified nutritional therapist. It seems that the goalposts keep moving. One day butter is bad for us, the next it is a superfood – and what is a superfood? I think nutrition is incredibly important and I didn't want to finish the book without including some words to help clear the confusion.

Liz Butler is Beauty Despite Cancer's nutritional therapist. Liz has worked in the field of cancer support for many years, and for most of those as head of nutrition for some very big and well-respected cancer charities. Kelly McCabe is a specialist oncology dietician at Leaders in Oncology Care (LOC) on Harley Street in London.

I asked Liz and Kelly to help.

Beginning Nutritional Therapy

I asked Liz if nutritional therapists work with clients as they go through treatment or if it is better to wait until treatment has finished.

The sooner a person with cancer can start working with a nutritional therapist, the better. Research shows that people who are well nourished have a more favourable outcome in terms of their cancer treatment, and the risk of side effects and complications is reduced. There is also evidence that a higher intake of certain nutrients can protect normal cells against some of the effects of cancer treatments.[39-43]

During treatment, nutritional needs may change, so it is advisable to continue receiving nutritional support at this time. Following treatment, needs may change again. A nutritional therapist can help a client to rebuild and strengthen their body.

There are some *don't do's* with regard to nutrition and cancer treatment; however, a nutritional therapist who is experienced in cancer care will use their knowledge and skill to design a programme that enhances rather than undermines the cancer treatment. It is important to remind patients of the things that they can do to help themselves. There are a lot of *can do's* in nutritional support for those living with cancer and beyond.

Nutritional therapy can be very beneficial for people living with cancer: survivors with a better nutritional status have fewer disease symptoms, a lower risk of treatment complications, greater longevity and an improved quality of life.[44-46] Nutritional therapy can also be very helpful for managing particular signs and symptoms of cancer and its treatments, for example fatigue and digestive problems.[47,48]

The power of nutritional therapy may extend beyond its physical benefits, as many people with cancer experience a psychological boost when they receive information and guidance on how to help themselves through positive lifestyle changes.[48]

Choosing a Therapist

If you live in the UK and are choosing a nutritional therapist, first of all make sure that the therapist is a member of the British Association for Applied Nutrition and Nutritional Therapy (BANT); this will demonstrate that they are trained to a high standard. Secondly, you should make sure that the nutritional therapist has several years of clinical experience in the field of cancer care and is confident in liaising with medical teams.

Once you have found a therapist who is well trained and experienced, the next thing is to ensure that you like their approach and manner of working with clients. The best way to do this is to have a preliminary meeting or chat on the phone.

The role of a nutritional therapist is to educate and advise clients on the most supportive diet and also, if appropriate, to give guidance on supplements. Most nutritional therapists will start by collecting information from the client using a health questionnaire. Recommendations will be given on the basis of a client's individual needs. Follow-up sessions are arranged, as these are necessary for providing further information, support and encouragement.

The client has the most difficult job – putting the advice given by the nutritional therapist into practice. However, the therapist and client will work together to decide which changes are a priority and how they should fit in with current lifestyle patterns. The changes should not be overwhelming or unsustainable.

Healthy Eating

As a specialist oncology dietician, Kelly McCabe works in a medical environment, helping patients with specific side effects of treatment, such as weight loss, weight gain, constipation and digestive issues.

Kelly finds that many patients want information about 'healthy eating' when treatment is over. Kelly has kindly given us her crash course, designed for those people who have recently completed treatment and for those who want to reduce their risk of cancer and improve their overall health.

- Avoid weight gain by maximising the nutritional value of your food. Stay clear of foods, e.g. sugar, containing 'empty calories', which offer no benefit.
- Aim for at least 75% of your diet to be of plant origin, i.e. fruits, vegetables, pulses, legumes, nuts and grains.
- Try to include at least two portions of fruits or vegetables in every meal, and at least one portion of pulses per day – e.g. add a handful of lentils to your soup or salad at lunch, or serve some beans with your evening meal.
- Aim to limit your red meat intake to once per week, and avoid salted or smoked meats altogether – this includes bacon, ham and chorizo. Fish, poultry, pulses, nuts, seeds, eggs or low-fat natural yoghurt are healthy alternatives.

- Have oily fish rich in omega-3, such as salmon, trout, sardines, mackerel, herring and fresh tuna, two to three times per week.
- Avoid sugary refined carbohydrates, including white bread; white pasta; and cakes, biscuits and sweets. Instead go for slow-release carbohydrates, such as oats, wholegrain pasta, wild rice, quinoa or sweet potato. Try to include a small, fist-sized portion with every meal. This will help you to be more in control of your energy levels and your appetite. You should experience fewer cravings as a result.
- Include healthy fats found in rapeseed oil, olive oil, nuts and avocado. Use them to replace other fats.

- Flavour your food with pepper, herbs, spices and citrus juice, rather than relying on salt.
- Minimise your alcohol intake and aim to have at least two consecutive alcohol-free days per week.
- It is really important for you to still enjoy your food. Follow the 80/20 rule: as long as you eat this way most of the time (80%), the occasional treats (20%) are fabulous, whether they be a glass of red wine, a fillet steak or a chocolate pudding.

Moving On

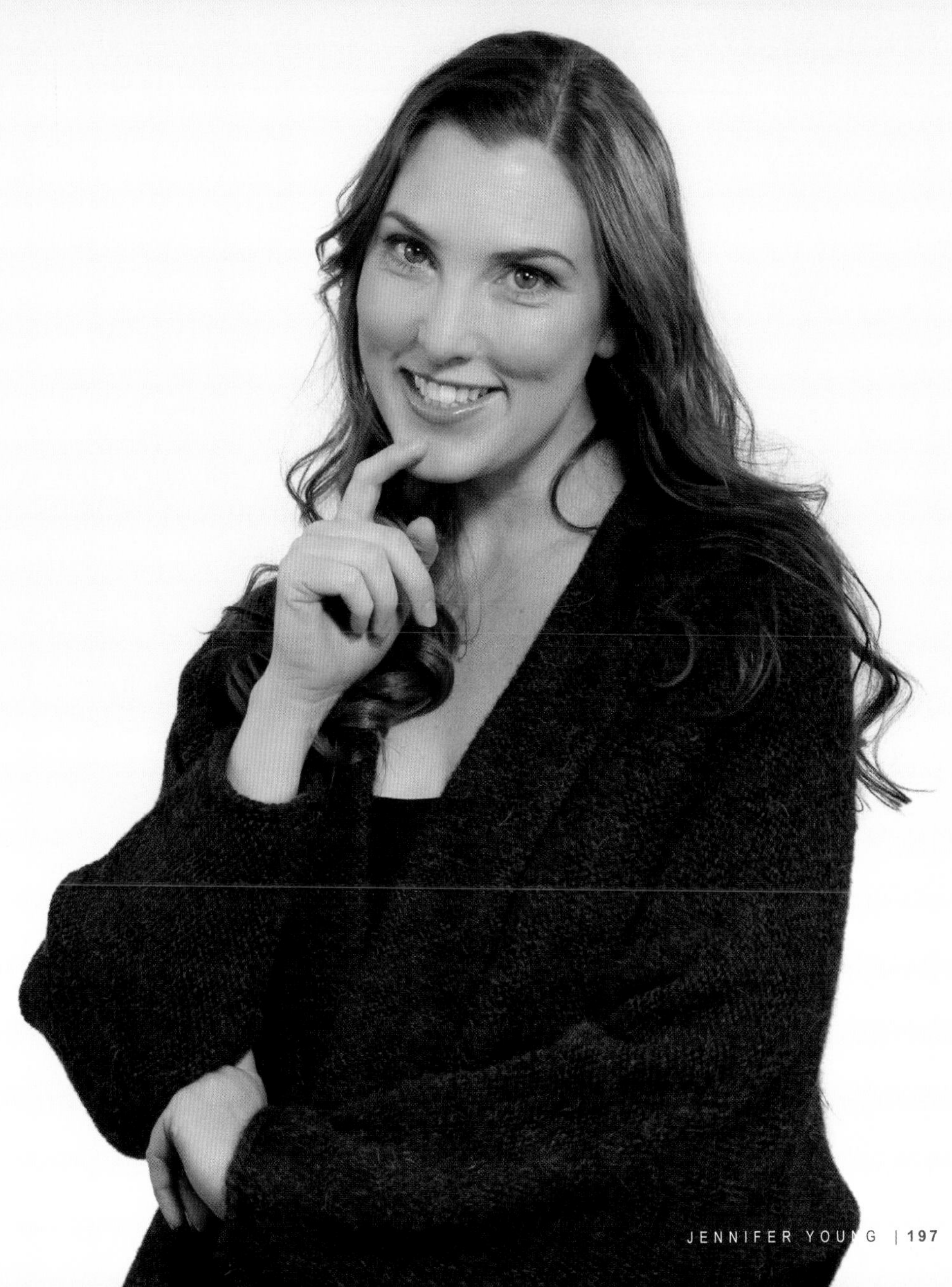

Moving On

And in the end, it's not the years in your life that count, it's the life in your years.

Life after Treatment

A cancer diagnosis and the subsequent treatment are all-consuming and can be terrifying. I meet so many people who are profoundly changed by the experience and don't know quite what to do afterwards. I cannot advise anyone on how to cope, but, thankfully, I know someone who can. Dr Mary Ivers, Head of Psychology at All Hallows College Dublin, conducts research into the lives and concerns of ex-patients. This is her advice.

So treatment is over and now you can go back to your life, or maybe you never left your life. For some, life is too changed and they cannot go back, so they begin creating a new life. There is no single common experience of 'life after cancer'. Everyone is different, and the physical and emotional experiences of cancer and its treatment will interact within each person to produce their 'life after cancer'. There is a growing body of knowledge aimed at helping make life after cancer a better-quality experience.[49-52]

Sometimes you may look back and wonder, did this really happen to you? You may feel violated, your life was threatened, the life you live was threatened, your identity was threatened.[53] To get to a good place after cancer, it is important to be able to maintain a sense of identity as you move through and beyond this rotten experience you have had. It is important to get comfortable with who you are now and to integrate the experience you have been through into your view of yourself and your future.[54] The common element is you – your past, your now and your future. After all the prodding and poking, it can be difficult to know who you are!

You may have to deal with some physical, psychological and emotional effects, as well as the social, financial and work-related consequences of having had cancer.[44, 45, 55] Sometimes people become dependent on others during treatment, have little belief that they have any control over what happens, have a low sense of self-worth and have difficulties envisioning a future.[56] A lady who participated in my research told me that she felt like she was 'set adrift' after her treatment ended. The picture she painted was of the line being cut, setting her loose from the safety of being in treatment to set sail into the 'uncharted territory'[43] of 'life after cancer'.

On top of that feeling you may have to deal with unexpected late-emerging side effects of treatment, including shock and distress about what has happened and fears and worries about the cancer returning – all while trying to get strong enough to feel you have some control over your future.[57] All of this is a big ask for someone who has had the stuffing knocked out of them!

If the experience has not really changed you or your life, that is wonderful! However, I don't think there are too many who are this lucky.[54] Any extremely stressful or traumatic experience, such as a cancer diagnosis, will usually force us to adapt and adjust our lives, and that fundamentally changes us.[56, 58]

The good news is that most people have a good life after cancer treatment. While many will have some health consequences, the research suggests that, for most cancers, the majority of people do not experience significant long-term effects.[50,59]

There is also some evidence that the experience of having cancer can have a positive impact, influencing some people to change direction as they seek to find meaning in the cancer experience by doing something different.[60] What you value in life may be quite different now as priorities change: you may change career, change your home life, spend more time with loved ones, aim to become healthier, focus on helping others – the list is endless.

'I had what I describe as a lucky encounter with cancer many years ago. When we have cancer the earth shifts beneath our feet. Nothing looks the same. Everything was up in the air, so I threw food up in the air too and added dietary changes to my determined recovery.

'I wouldn't now be running a vegan and gluten-free restaurant if I hadn't had that experience all of those years ago.'

Magdalena Chávez, owner, El Piano, York

Prepare Yourself

In recent years more information and assistance have become available to help people navigate their way through 'life after cancer'. Understanding the issues that people have to deal with as a result of their cancer experience is helping health care teams to modify treatments and provide resources that help people deal with those issues.

So what can help you manage the move forwards? How can you take care of yourself so that you can have a good 'life after cancer'? There are no simple answers, but there are a few key actions that can help.

One thing you can do is to prepare yourself – you want to avoid being taken by surprise. Gather information about the common issues affecting people with your type of cancer and ask questions when you see your oncologist; share this information with your family and friends.[61] Having the necessary information will reduce the stress associated with unexpected side effects. In the midst of being told don't do this and don't do that, try to remember to ask: 'What can I do?'

Your Support Network

While it is all about you – your past, your now and your future – this does not mean you have to go it alone. One of the most important resources available to you is your support network. Good-quality social support is good for your health.[58, 62, 63] Going through cancer will put a strain on your relationships. It is important to work on surrounding yourself with people who are good for you, who help you feel safe and who encourage you.

Sometimes getting involved with a support group is just what you need. Having people who understand what it is like is a great way of helping you feel that you aren't alone. But it is not everyone's cup of tea! Remember, you can get support in many places, including the online community.

Once your treatment is over, and you look like you are 'back to normal', your friends and family may not understand that the cancer experience is not completely behind you and they may expect too much from you. It is important to talk to them and show them the information you have gathered about living after cancer and ask them to help you. Working on strengthening the good relationships in your life is good for your physical and mental health.

It is important to know yourself and admit it if you feel you aren't managing very well. Sometimes we cope by not acknowledging the situation we are in, and when we finally ask for help we realise that we should have asked sooner. This avoidance coping is not very helpful in the long run.

It is best, if you can, to acknowledge the traumatic experience you have been through and the worries you now have. Seek information and support to help you work through it. This is not easy, as there can be a lot to deal with and you may feel overwhelmed. This is another reason to surround yourself with a safety net of good people. Don't suffer in silence – there is a lot of help out there.

If you have pain, are anxious or have other symptoms that make you miserable, tell your oncologist or your GP. If you get the opportunity to go to a survivorship programme or a rehabilitation programme, take it. Such programmes often focus on giving a lot of useful information, as well as reducing stress and advising about living a healthier lifestyle. All of these will help you have a better quality of life.

Coping with Life after Cancer

One of the most challenging aspects of life after cancer is a lack of confidence in yourself and your future. This can be fuelled by your usual way of viewing the world and by fears about cancer recurrence. There is no denying that having cancer and going through treatment will change your outlook on life. Many people feel hopeless and helpless, as they are overwhelmed by the whole experience.

We know that having a more optimistic or hopeful outlook is a real benefit. This is not about pretending that everything is OK but

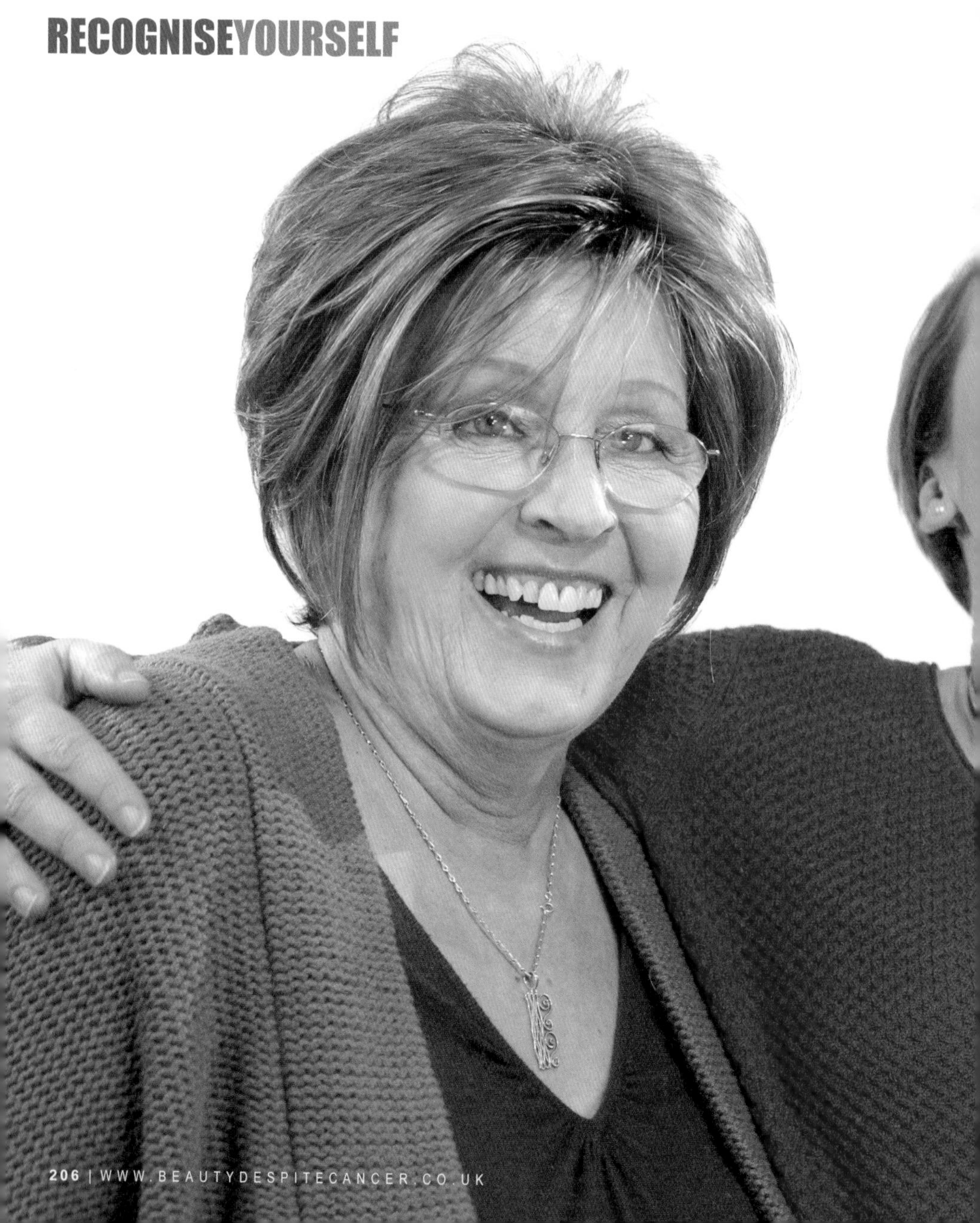

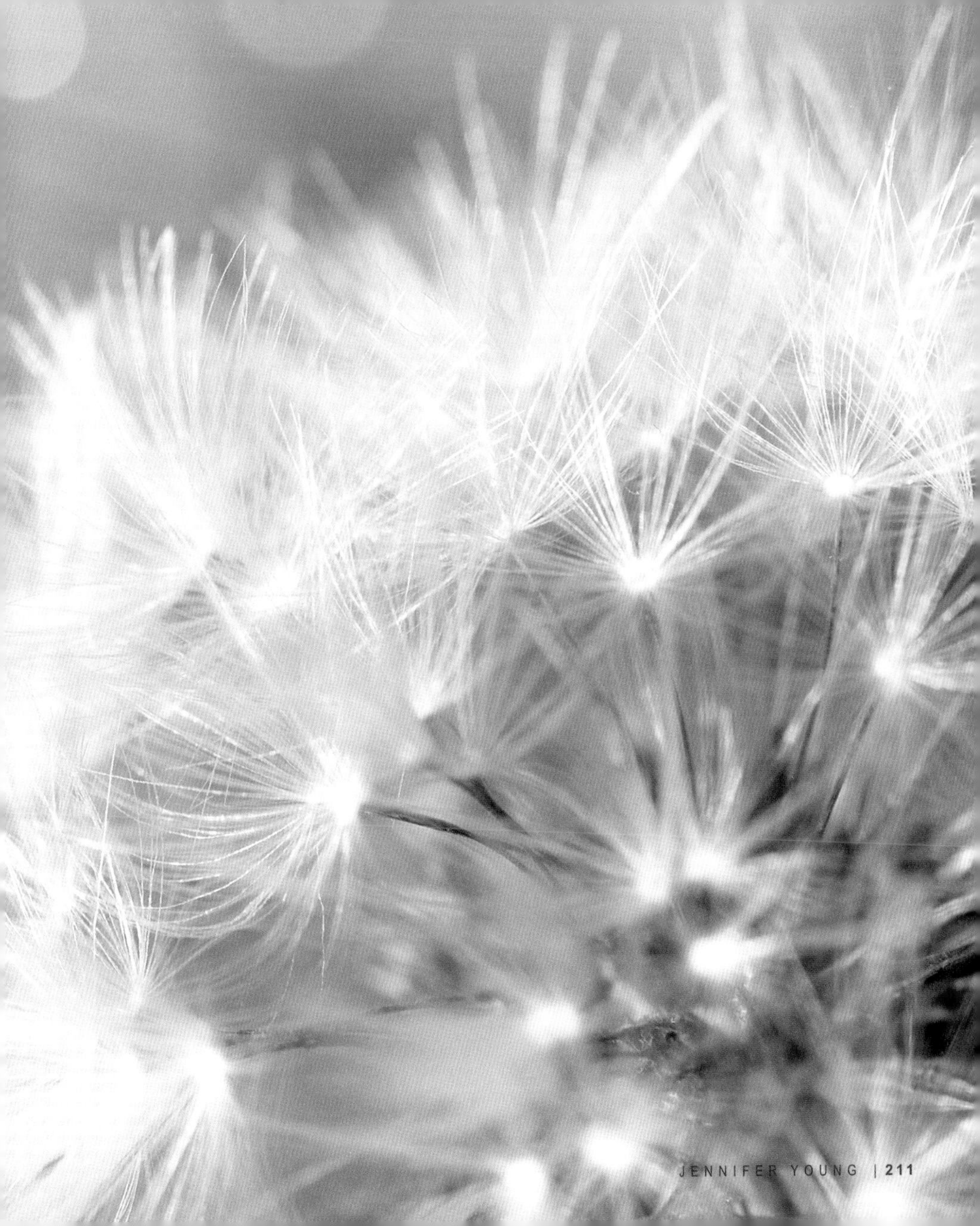

Appendix 1
Photo Shoot

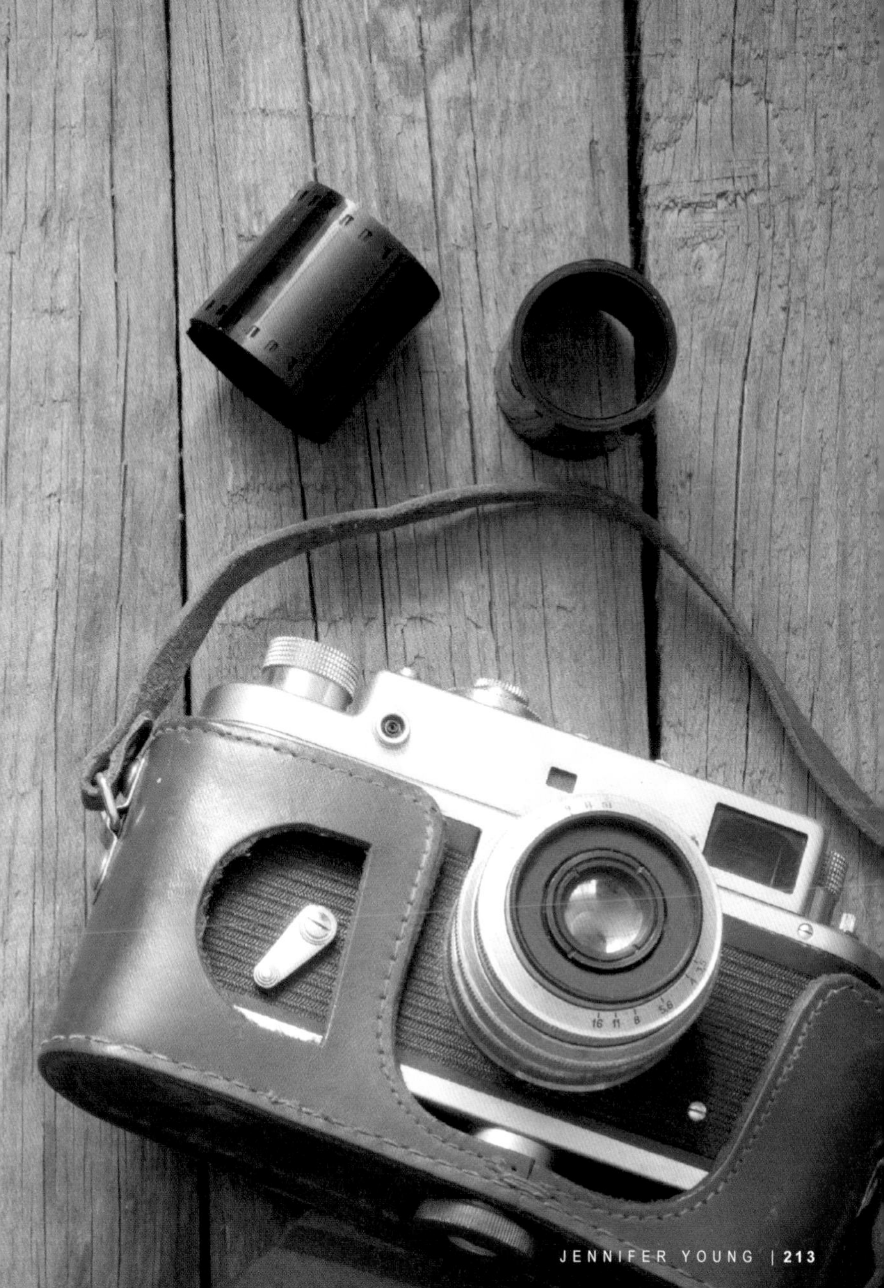

I think that the photographs in this book are amazing, truly outstanding and completely unique. They are here because of the kindness, generosity and hard work (really hard work) of the people featured in the following pages.

Everyone gave their time and considerable expertise free of charge as they wanted to show those living with cancer and beyond that it is possible to recognise yourself, to love the reflection that you see in the mirror and to step out with confidence.

Women don't stop being women when they are diagnosed with cancer and, thanks to the generosity of the people that you will meet in the next few pages, you can see that you can continue to be a woman and not only that, the fabulous-looking woman that you always were.

My love and thanks to all involved on that wonderful day.

Claudio Sardone

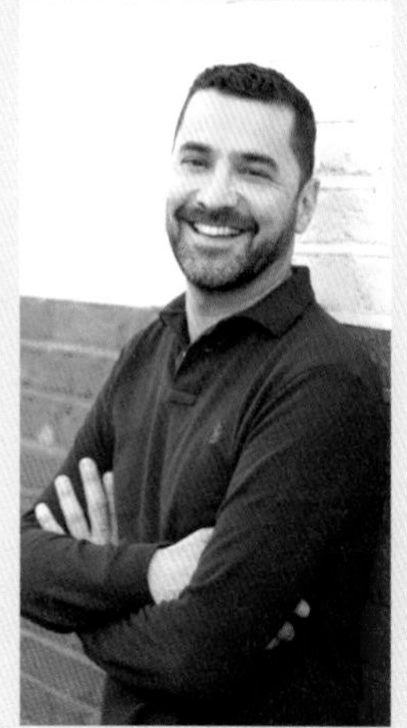

Born in Rome, where he studied photography and filming. Photographer, TV producer and director, Claudio has dedicated over 20 years to capturing and creating momentums in both still and moving images. Claudio has worked on countless projects including working with MTV in London, LA and Milan.

Zuzana Markova

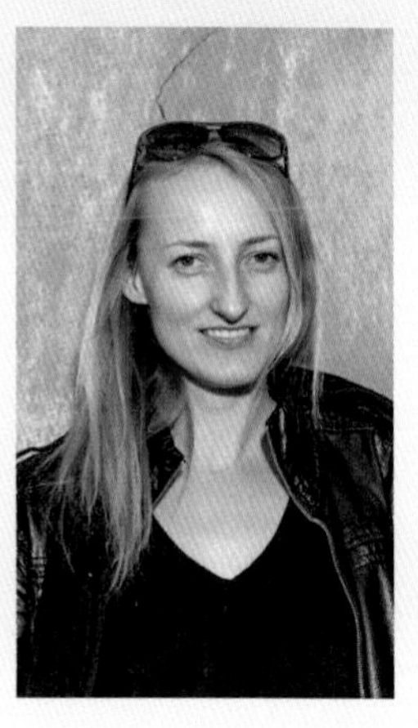

Born in Ostrava, Czech Republic. Zuzana has studied film and cinematography. She has a successful career in the film and TV industry, currently working for AMC Networks broadcasting and producing award-winning series such as *Breaking Bad*.

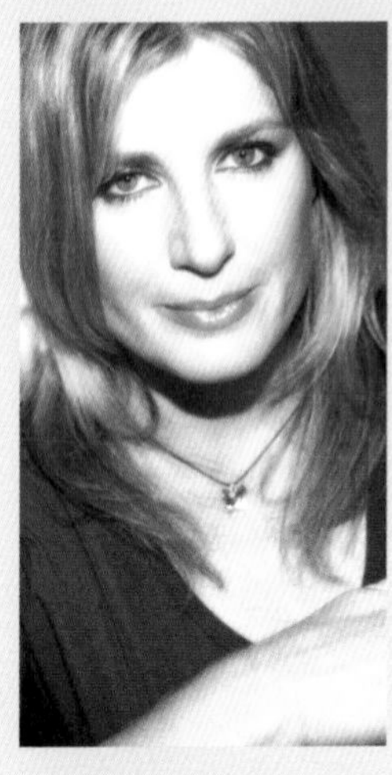

Melissa Lackersteen

Melissa wanted to be a make-up artist from a young age and studied Specialised Make-Up at London College of Fashion.

Melissa's work includes *Son of the Pink Panther, Four Weddings and a Funeral, Gladiator, Star Wars, The Phantom Menace, Casino Royale, Tomb Raider, the Harry Potter films and Game of Thrones.*

www.makeupmatters.co.uk

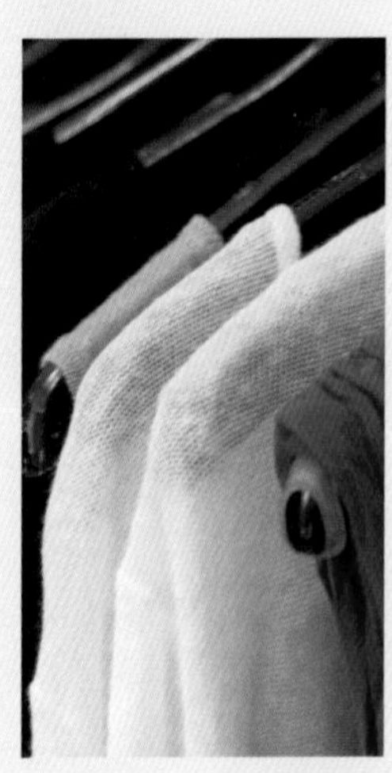

WALL London

Established in 1997, WALL London clothing is designed for women to look as great as they feel.

WALL London is not a mass-market brand; they care about where goods come from and who makes them. WALL's clothes are made to the absolute best quality they can be.

Be kind to your body with WALL.

www.wall-london.com

Natalie Fox

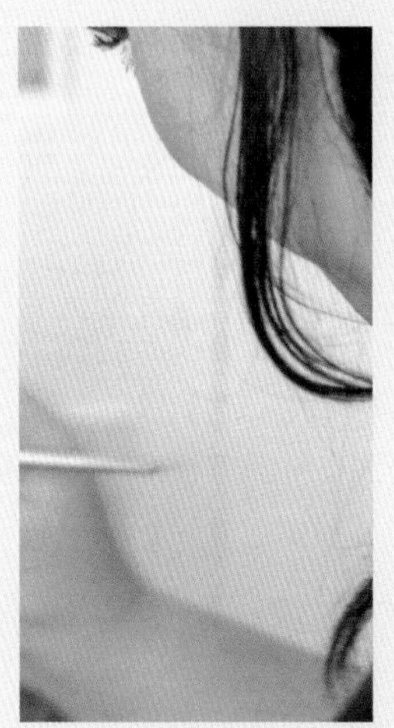

Make-up artist Natalie Fox has worked on exciting projects such as London Fashion Week; fashion shows for the V&A; editorials for fashion magazines; and commercial images for brands, *This Morning* and *Loose Women.*

Natalie is now training in wigs and assisting in the West End on shows such as *Les Miserables and The Lion King*.

Rosie Willoughby

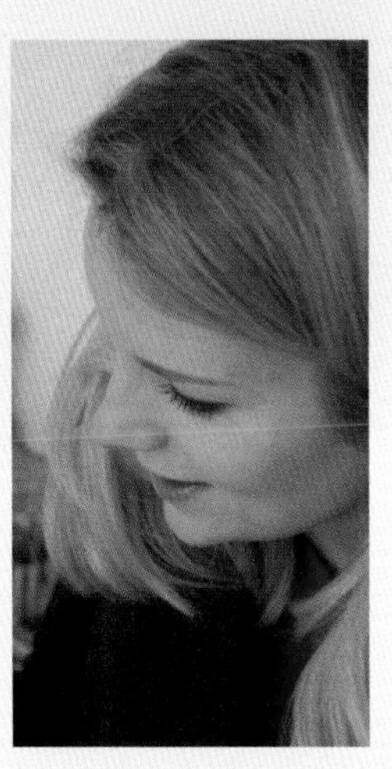

Located in London, Paris trained and with nearly a decade's experience in make-up. Rosie has worked with *Vogue, Elle, Harper's Bazaar,* L'Oreal and Elle McPherson, and has contributed to the creation of a limited range for MAC and a training program for Chanel make-up artists.

Rosie is part of the appearance team at LOC, Harley Street.

http://rosiewilloughby.com

http://www.theloc.com

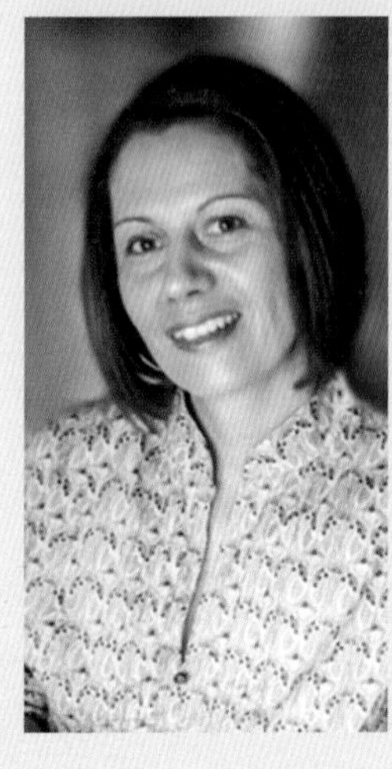

Claire Featherstone

After working as a clothing importer and, later, director for a large UK business, Claire set up Featherstone Frocks. Claire's clients told her of the need for 'high-end' headwear, and 'Chemo Headwear' was born.

Claire lost both of her parents to cancer when she was in her twenties.

www.chemoheadwear.co.uk

www.featherstonefrocks.com

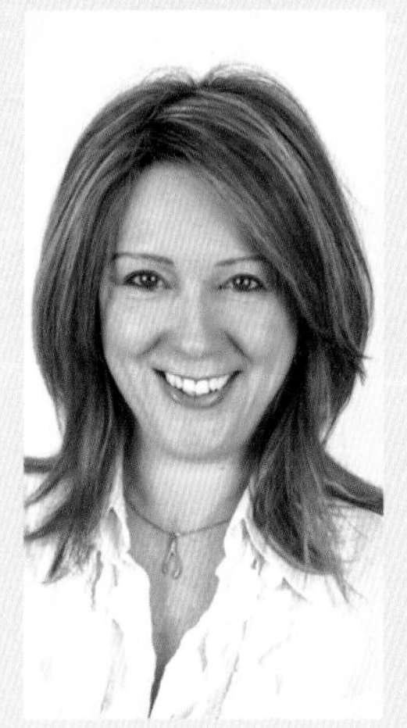

Audrey McLarn Ball

Audrey Ball is a London-based hair loss expert and image consultant. Drawing on her 30-year hair loss journey, she is able to meet the practical and emotional needs of those experiencing hair loss.

Audrey uses her extensive knowledge of the wig and hair replacement industry to guide her clients through the practical and emotional challenges of losing hair.

www.esteemwigs.co.uk

Talena Zatrieb

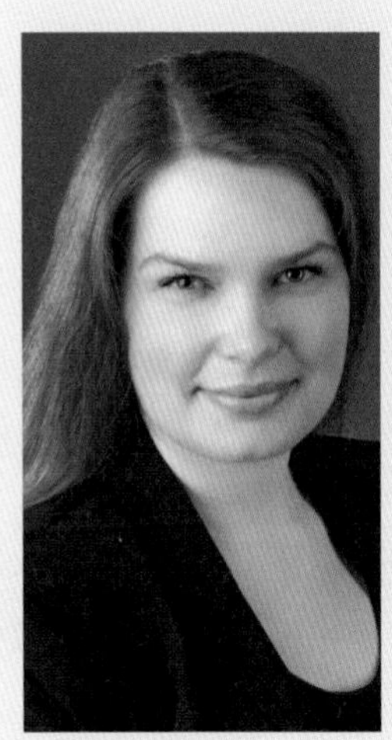

Whilst working as an intern with Rebecca Goodyear PR, Talena was invited to experience a photo shoot, joining Jennifer and the team on their big day.

Talena was an invaluable team member as hers was the extra pair of hands that everyone needed, at all times. As a consequence, Talena went home exhausted and happy at the end of a very special day.

Keating Mary

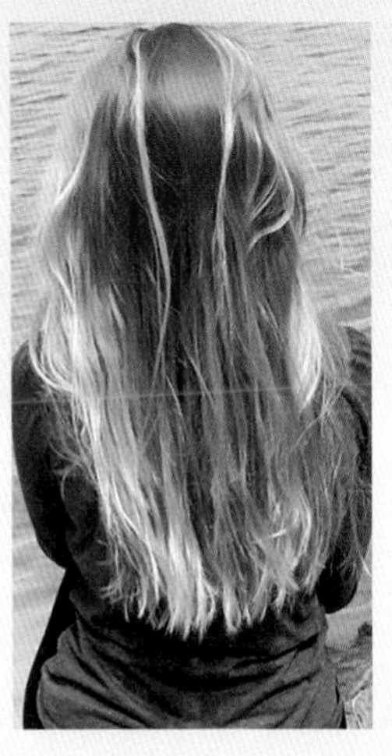

Keating Mary, photographer and social media manager, captured our 'behind-the-scenes images'. She also ensured that our activities were shared on Beauty Despite Cancer and Jennifer Young's social media platforms.

This was Keating Mary's first experience of a professional shoot and her first commission. We are sure that it won't be her last.

Appendix 2

Should I Tell the Children?

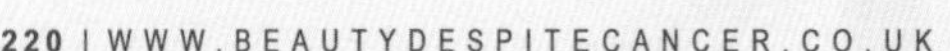

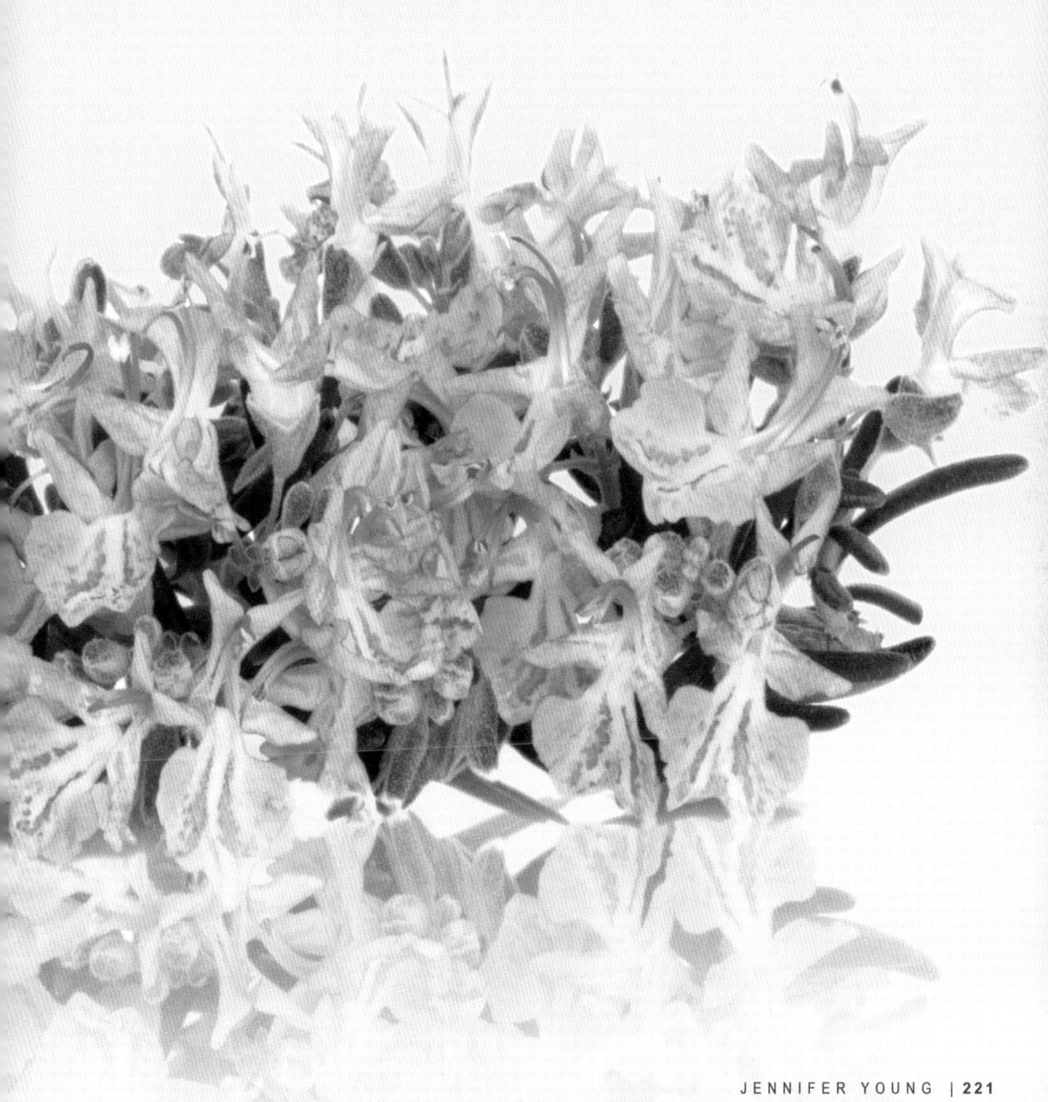

We all want to do what is best for our children; we protect them from harm. You know your children need support, but how do you support them?

You may feel the need to protect them from your hair loss.

Lyndsay Dobson, the family therapist at East Cheshire Hospice, works with children who have a parent undergoing treatment for cancer. Having worked as a family therapist in a hospice environment for over ten years, she is constantly amazed and humbled by the strength of the children with whom she works.

Lyndsay suggests that you approach issues such as hair loss with honesty and in a way that your child will understand – include your children:

'You know your child better than anyone – be guided by them. Sometimes that is scary. If you take the risk of allowing your child into what is a scary and uncertain place, often they will surprise you by their resilience and ability to cope.

‘Children are far more perceptive than we realise. If we don’t tell them the truth, they can make up some scary stories for themselves.

‘Children, especially young ones, are very self-orientated; the world revolves around them. If mum and dad are arguing or crying, or if the house seems tense and scared, they often think: “It must be my fault.”’

If you don’t explain what is happening, children can make up their own explanations. If we don’t tell them the truth, or if we try to hide things from them, they learn not to trust, and that is scary for a child.

If you include your children, be honest in response to the questions they pose; that way, they will know they can still trust you, talk to you, or come to you for cuddles if they need to. Instead of being alone in the dark, they are in it with you, holding your hand.

Communicating with children can be difficult. Lyndsay has some advice:

‘Find a way of talking to your child that works for you as a family – use stories or art, or sit and talk for a few moments. Come back to the

subject later – young children can't take in a lot of information at one time. They need to be given information in small chunks, over and over again. Play it out with dolls or puppets or relate it to a storyline on TV. The ways you can do this are endless and as unique as your family and child.

'Never force information on a child – if they don't want to know, that's OK. Never underestimate how much your child can take in and hear while seemingly ignoring you and playing in the corner!'

‘We didn’t know how to prepare our daughter for my wife’s hair loss. There were no rules. We just did our best. Our three-year-old M took it all in her stride and became mummy’s scarf stylist. M would decide which scarf went with which outfit, and there was rarely a day when my wife decided on headwear for herself.’

Pete Wallroth, founder of Mummy’s Star

Appendix 3

Wig Care

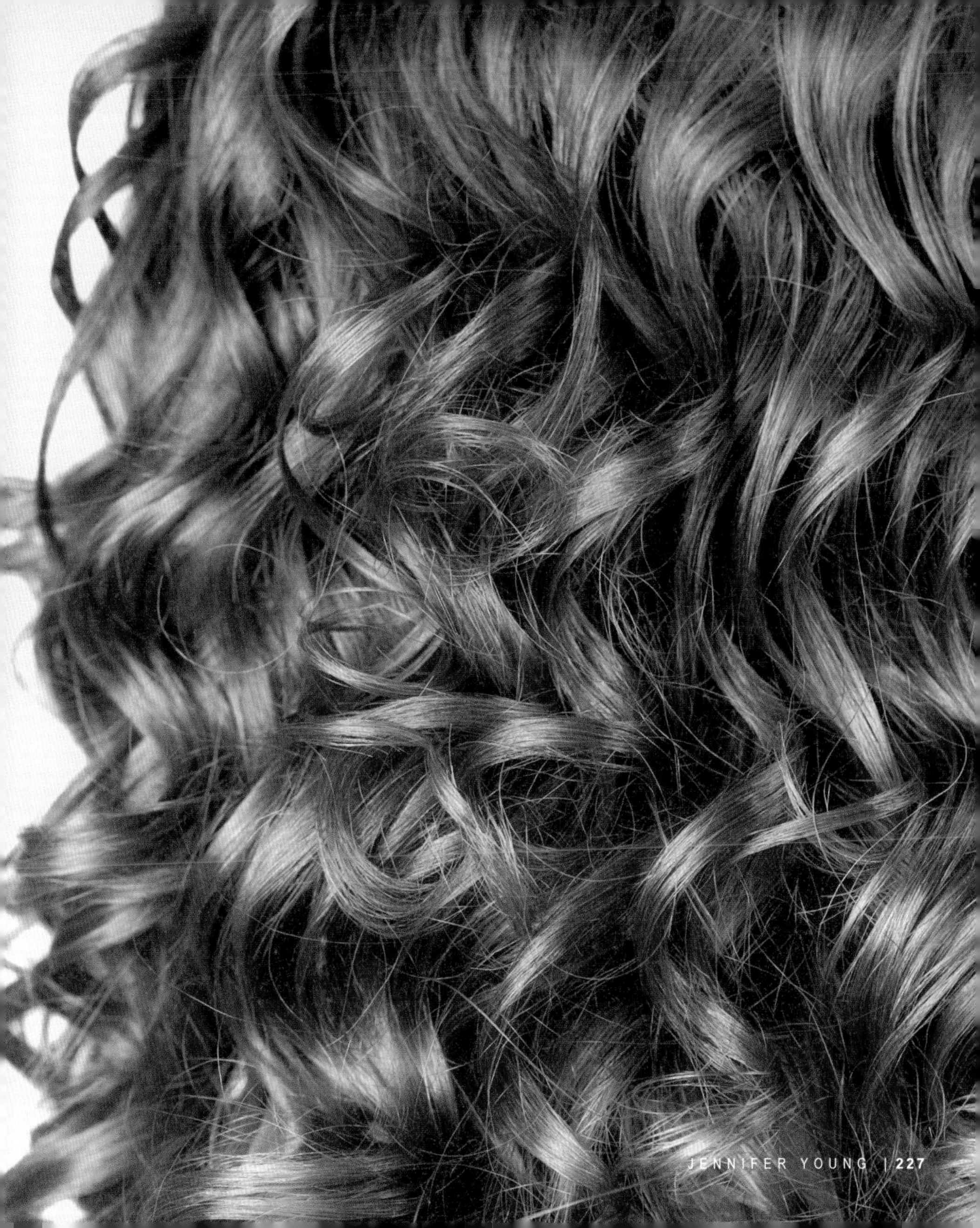

Wig Care

Washing/conditioning instructions:

- Use cold/tepid water from your shower – not warm water.
- Hold the wig in one hand at the crown.
- Douse the wig on the outside first until thoroughly wet.
- Turn the wig inside out and douse inside.
- Return to the outside.
- Take a good quantity of shampoo and work it through the wig evenly, from the roots to the tips.
- Avoid scrubbing – simply use the fingers to work the shampoo through, from roots to tips.
- Leave the shampoo in for a few minutes and then rinse clear.
- Repeat the process with a conditioner.
- Leave the conditioner in for 5–10 minutes and then rinse clear.

- Hold the wig at the crown and shake lightly.
- Fold the wig into a towel and pat on a flat surface. Leave for a few minutes.
- Remove the towel and lie the wig flat to dry for a few hours.
- During this time, turn the wig into different positions to help the drying process.
- When the wig is completely dry, place it on a wig stand or block.
- Brush/comb through and style.

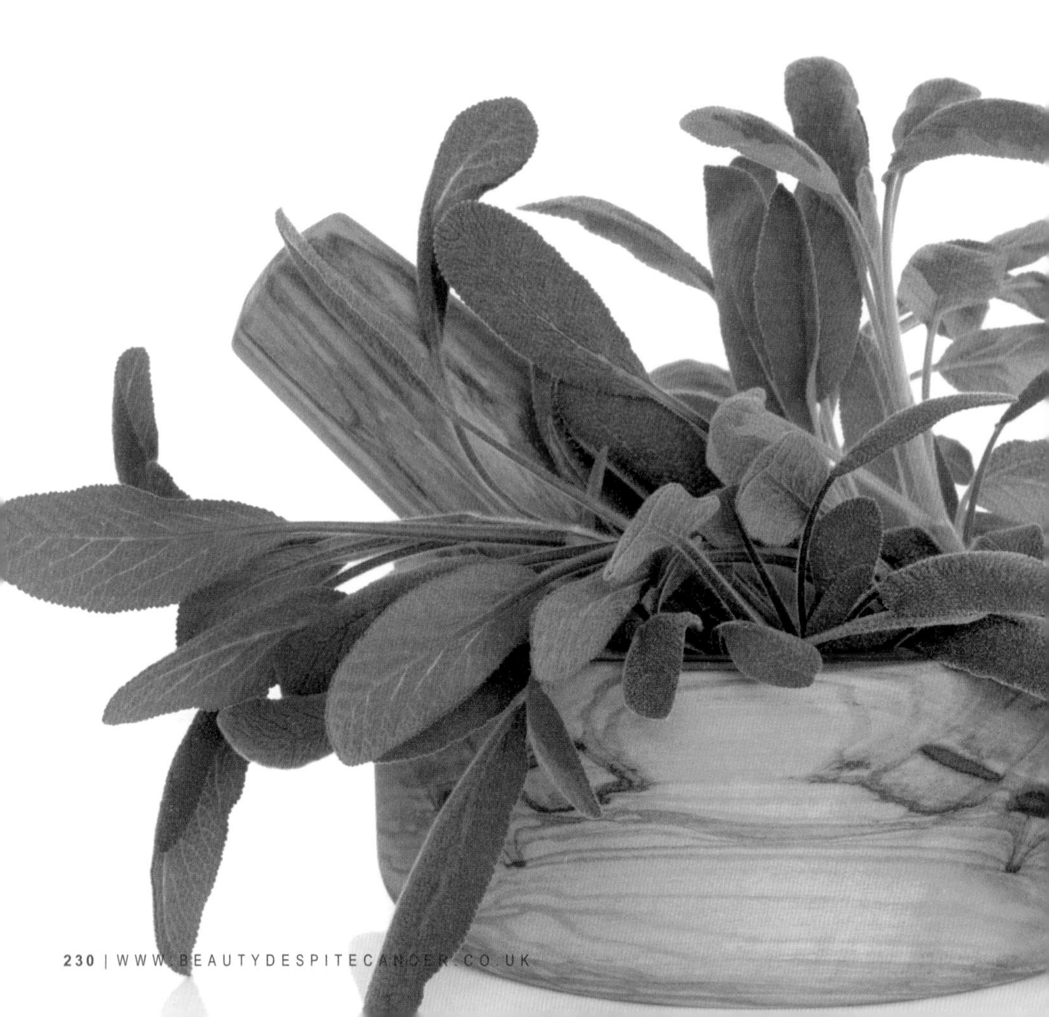

Appendix 4
Choosing a Complementary and Beauty Therapist

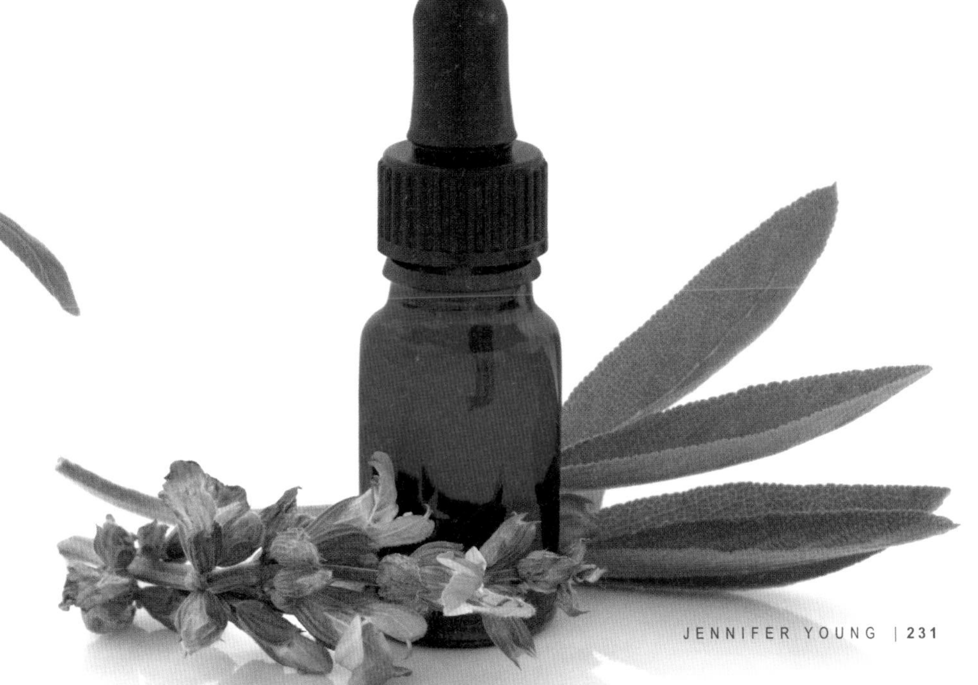

You can gain great and well-documented[21] benefits from complementary and beauty therapists as you go through treatment. Lots of hospitals and support centres offer these services.

Many women prefer to receive complementary and beauty therapies outside of what they perceive to be a medical setting. Some, however, are unable to access the services that they require. For example, few hospitals offer holistic facials through their complementary therapy departments, yet many women suffering from skin changes during treatment feel that a facial would benefit them.[67]

When deciding upon your therapists, there are some things that you should think about.

Training and Membership of the Appropriate Professional Body

A good therapist should be able to talk you through their qualifications and put you in touch with the organisations that provide accreditation and/or with professional bodies. Membership of such bodies is usually voluntary, but I strongly suggest that you choose therapists who have joined their professional body.

The therapist should also have experience of working with clients as they go through treatment. Specialist training courses in, for example, oncology massage or facials are essential. I would advise against allowing someone without specialist training and qualification to work with you.

Standards of Hygiene

I am aware of the fact that I keep mentioning this, but it is important – you are likely to have a compromised immunity.

Standards of hygiene within the salon environment are a good indicator of the thought that therapists have put into the 'control of cross infection' – in other words, the steps that they have taken to ensure that you don't pick up any bugs from their previous clients, the therapist themselves or the salon environment.

Therapists with specialist knowledge will be able to reassure you that they have taken the steps necessary to protect you. The steps are not onerous, but they do need to be taken. They are in addition to those usually mandatory.

Again, appropriately trained and responsible therapists will not carry out treatments that are unsuitable. For example, manicures and pedicures should be modified for you. Invasive procedures, such as semi-permanent make-up, are usually inappropriate, and medical consent should always be sought.

Talking to Your Medical Team

A good therapist will always talk to your medical team; it is part of the training on many specialist courses. Never work with a therapist who is not comfortable liaising with your medical team.

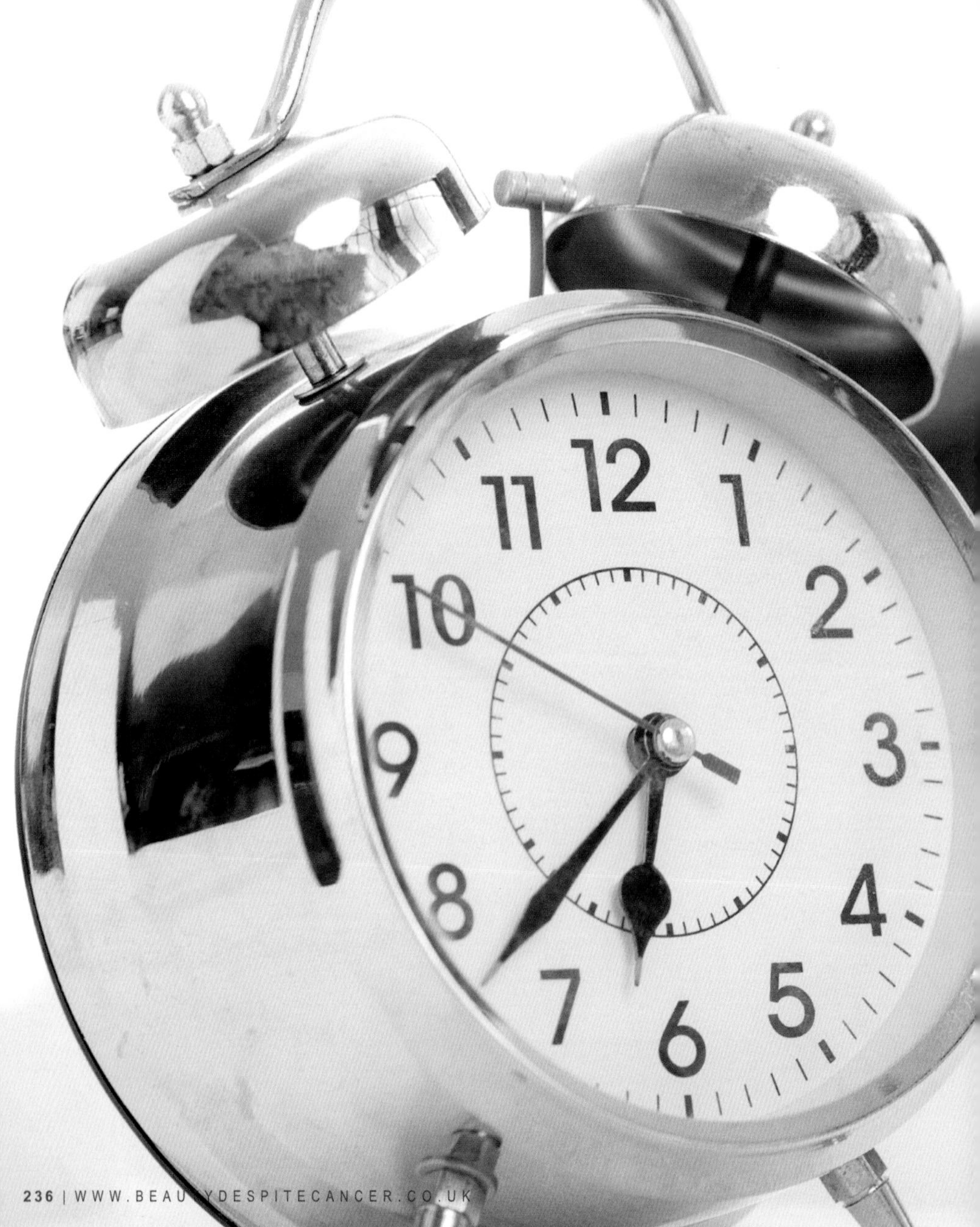

Appendix 5
Sleep Tips

Provided by Pat Duckworth, Harley Street Master NLP Practitioner and cognitive hypnotherapist.

Keep a sleep journal:

- A sleep journal can identify patterns that aid good sleep or result in poor sleep.

Make your bedroom a sleep haven:

- Remove the TV, mobile phone and computers.
- Make sure the room is dark, cool, quiet and well ventilated.
- Invest in a good mattress and comfortable pillows.
- Use bed linen and bed clothes made of natural fibres.

Plan a calming bedtime routine:

- Lower the light levels as the evening progresses.
- Avoid TV programmes, books and computer games that stress or overexcite you.
- Take a warm bath or shower.

- Watch an amusing TV programme.
- Listen to soft music.
- Have a warm, non-caffeinated drink.
- Read an engaging book or magazine.

Once in bed, practise techniques to soothe your mind:

- Breathe out for longer than you breathe in, by counting to five as you breathe in and to seven as you breathe out. This triggers the parasympathetic system and relaxes the body.
- To relax the body, beginning at the toes, tense them and relax them. Flex the feet and relax them. Move up your body, tensing and relaxing your muscles. When your attention moves to your head, clench and relax your jaw. Then imagine your cheeks, and finally the top of your head, being gently massaged.
- You may find it easier to calm your mind if you listen to some soothing music as you move towards sleep.

Practise the three-minute break (as described by Professor Mark Williams, Oxford University):

The first minute, notice what is going on in your head – notice your thoughts, without trying to change them or judge them.For the second minute, move your attention to your breathing. Notice the sensation of it, the sound of it, the rhythm of it. Don't try to control it – just follow the breath. If your attention wanders, bring it back.

For the final minute, expand your attention to your whole body and notice any sensations in your feet, torso, face, arms, etc. Notice them, without judging or trying to change them. Leave out or let go of any emotions associated with those sensations.

If you are experiencing an uncomfortable sensation (e.g. hotness, nausea or itchiness):

- Close your eyes and imagine a control room in your mind. There are controls here for all of the functions of your body.
- Go into the control room and find the control panel for the sensation you are experiencing. Notice where the indicator on the control panel is pointing.
- Turn down the control for the sensation you are experiencing. For example, if you are hot, turn the control from 'hot' towards 'cool', or if you are nauseous, from 'nauseous' towards 'comfortable'.
- When the sensation has diminished, move away from the panel and leave the control room.

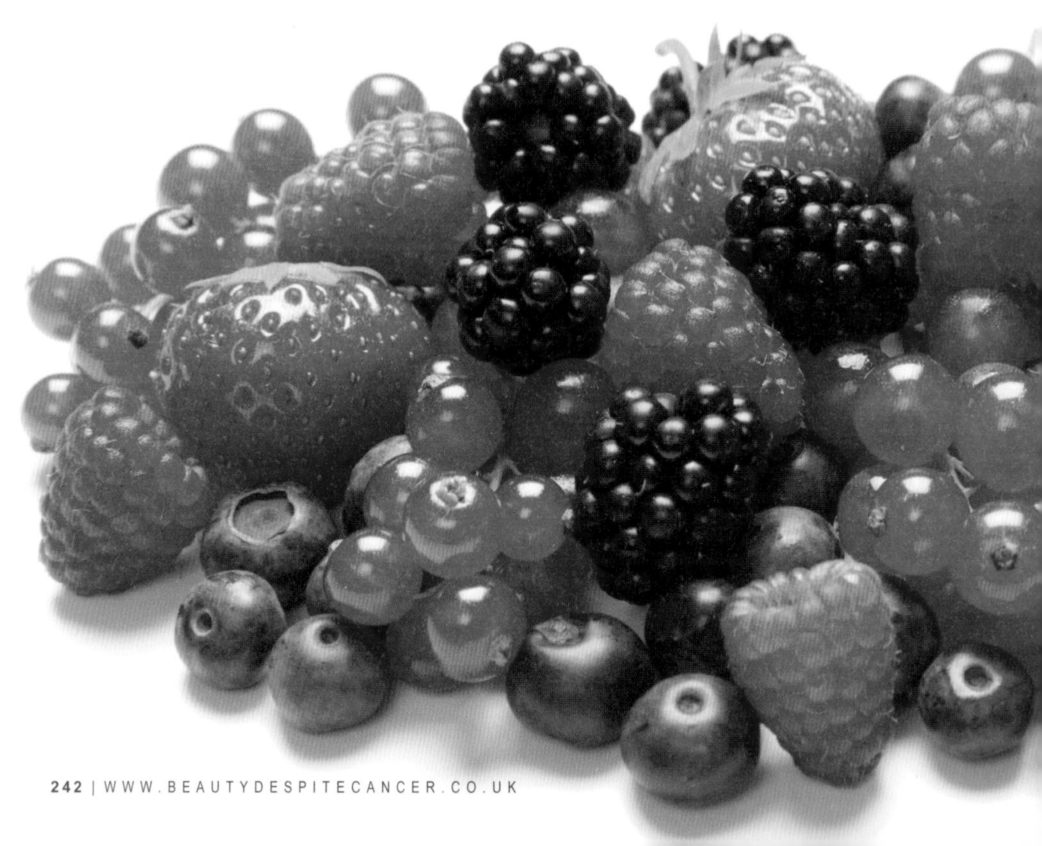

Appendix 6
Anti-ageing Recipes

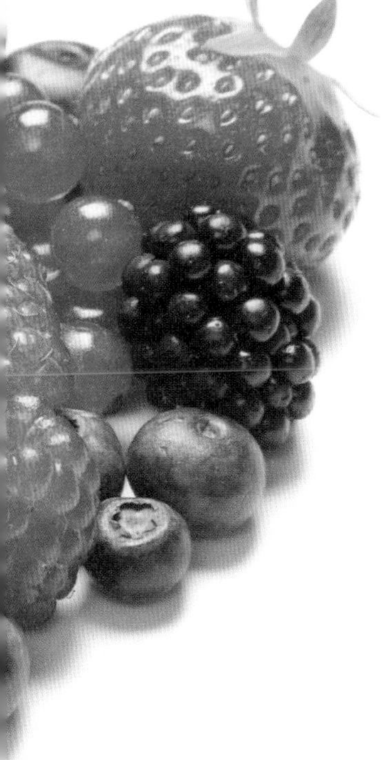

Asian-style Salad Leaves

Ingredients

- 2 heads radicchio, cut into quarters
- 2 heads romaine lettuce, sliced
- 2 heads endive, cut into quarters
- 6 spring onions, cut into large pieces
- 3 tbsp sherry vinegar
- 2 tbsp soy sauce
- 1 tbsp grated fresh ginger
- 2 cloves garlic, chopped
- 2 tbsp smooth peanut butter
- 1 finely chopped chilli (or more depending on your taste)
- 2 tsp honey
- 1 tsp toasted sesame oil
- 6 tbsp light olive oil
- Small bunch coriander
- Salt and freshly ground black pepper

For the vinaigrette, put the vinegar, soy sauce, ginger, garlic, peanut butter, chilli, honey and sesame oil in a blender and blend until smooth. With the motor running, slowly add the olive oil until the mixture is emulsified. If the vinaigrette is too thick add a little warm water. Season the vinaigrette with salt and pepper.

To prepare the leaves, brush them with oil, and season with salt and pepper. Grill them under a high heat until they are light golden brown and arrange them on a plate.

Drizzle the leaves with the vinaigrette, and garnish with the spring onions and chopped coriander.

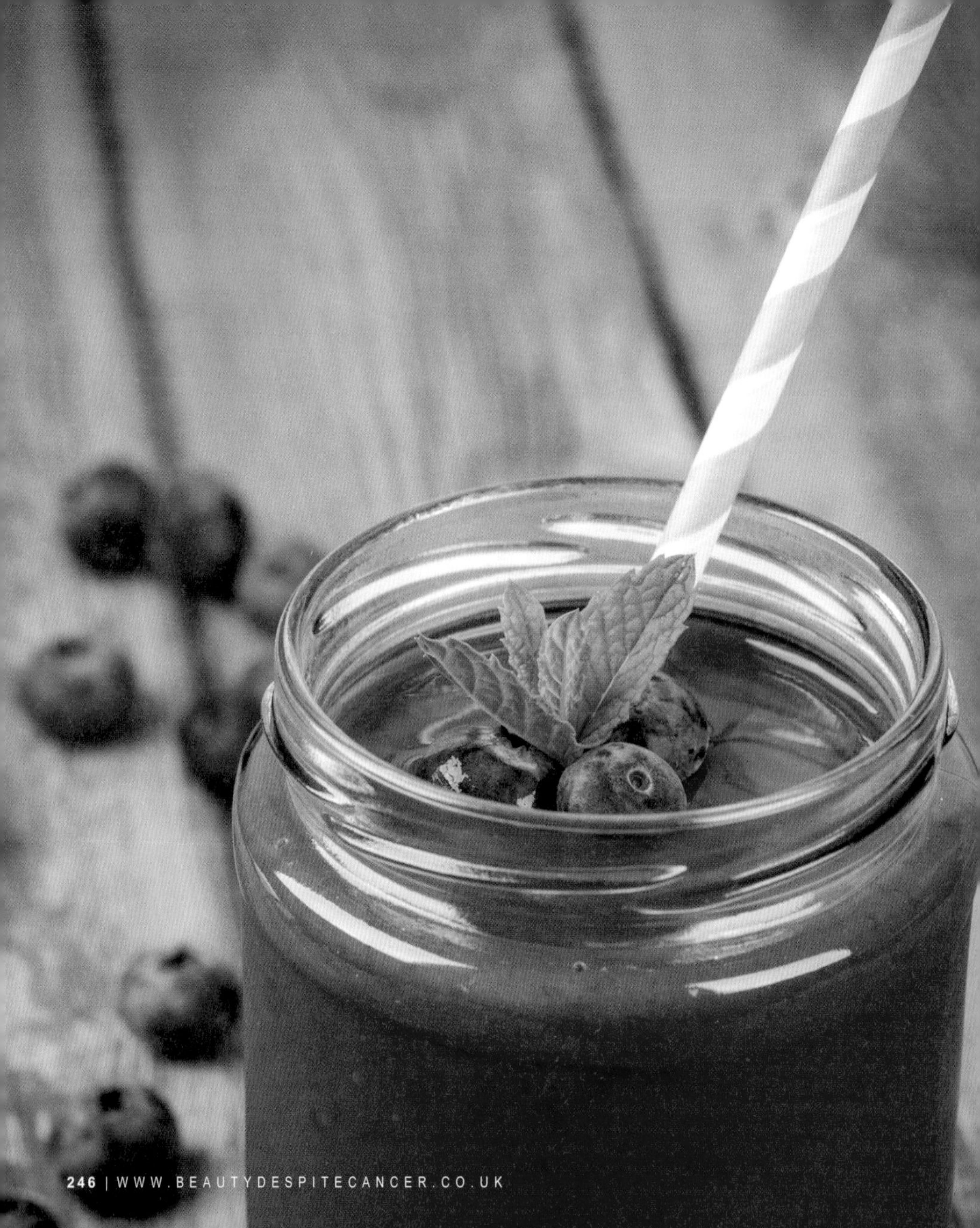

Blueberry and Avocado Smoothie

Ingredients

- 1 tbsp almonds
- Half an avocado
- 100 g blueberries
- 1 tsp raw honey
- 1 tsp raw cocoa powder
- 1 tsp maca powder
- Enough oat milk to produce the correct consistency

Grind the almonds to a fine powder in a blender or seed grinder. Combine with the other ingredients and blend until smooth in a blender.

Recipes kindly provided by Liz Butler of Body Soul Nutrition.

Appendix 7
What is a Cream?

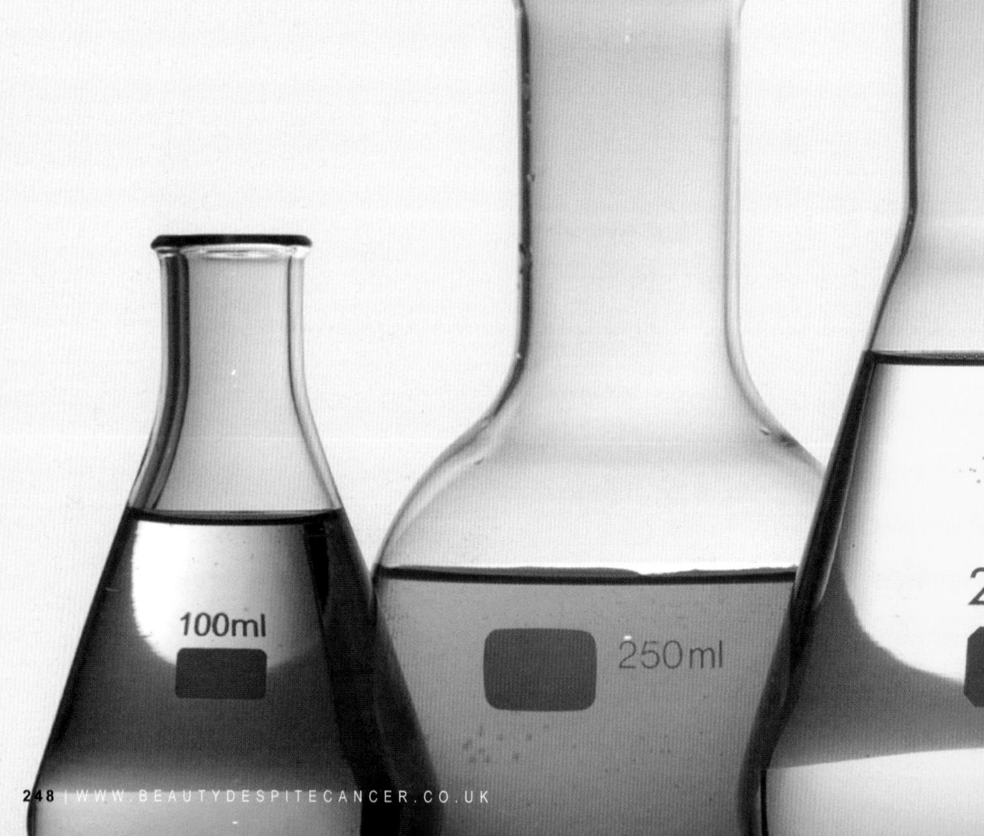

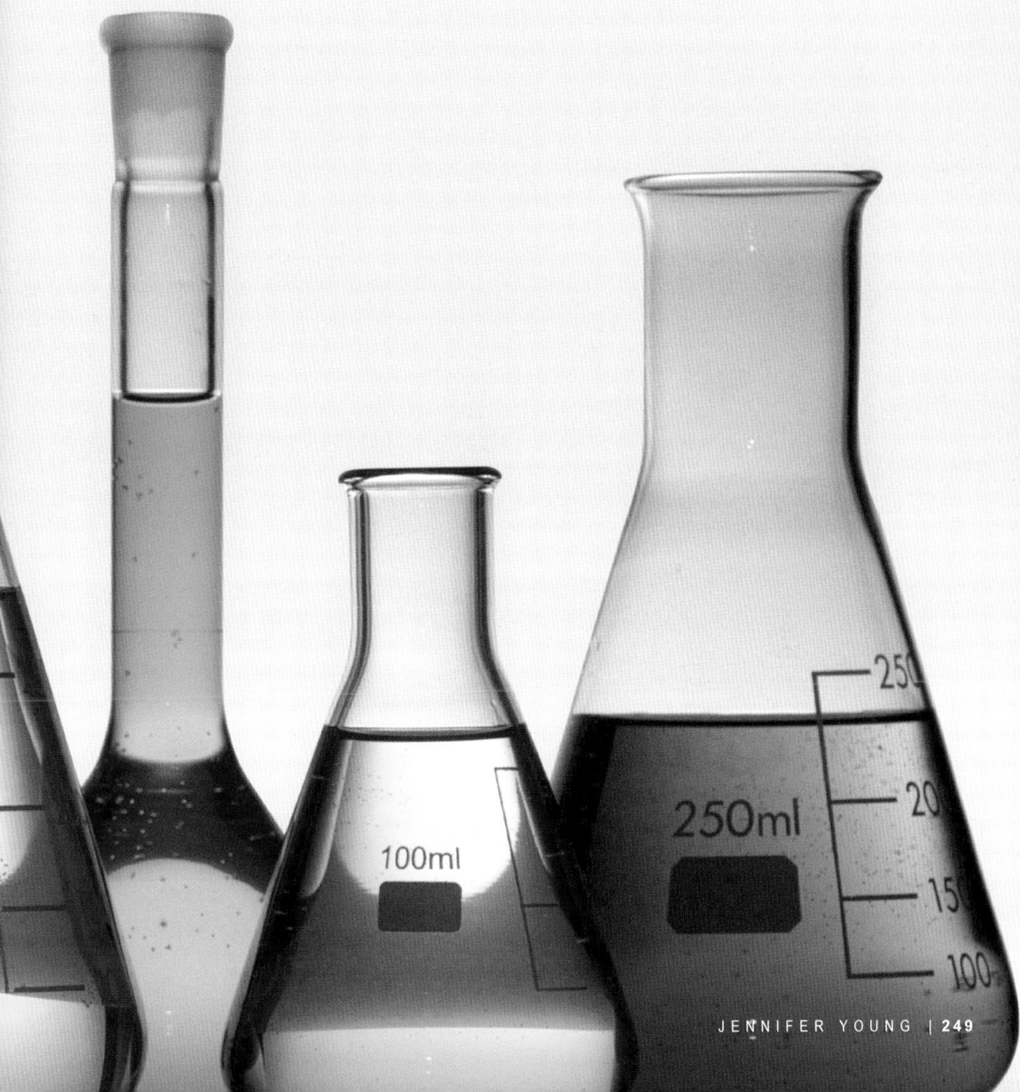
100ml
250ml
250
200
150
100

Clients often ask me why I never recommend cream or a lotion.

The Defiant Beauty Collections do not contain creams or lotions as our clients have very sensitive skin.

Creams and lotions are complex formulations that are, in essence, a mixture of oil and water. As oil and water don't mix naturally, emulsifying agents have to be added to the formulation, along with preservatives, conditioners, colours, pH adjusters and other ingredients to turn the unpleasant mix of oil, water and emulsifying agents into a light, white, fluffy cream or lotion that smells and feels good.

Creams and lotions cannot be made without using a large number of ingredients. As those living with cancer and beyond often have sore, sensitive, dry, itchy and damaged skin, we keep the number of ingredients in our products to a minimum – no creams or lotions. Oil-based products such as balms contain far fewer ingredients, thus reducing the likelihood of a reaction.

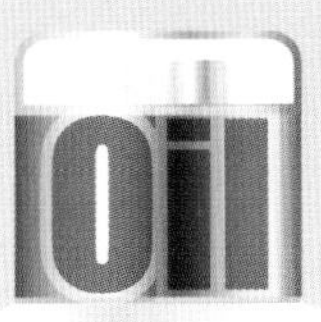

Oil

Natural Stabiliser

Cream

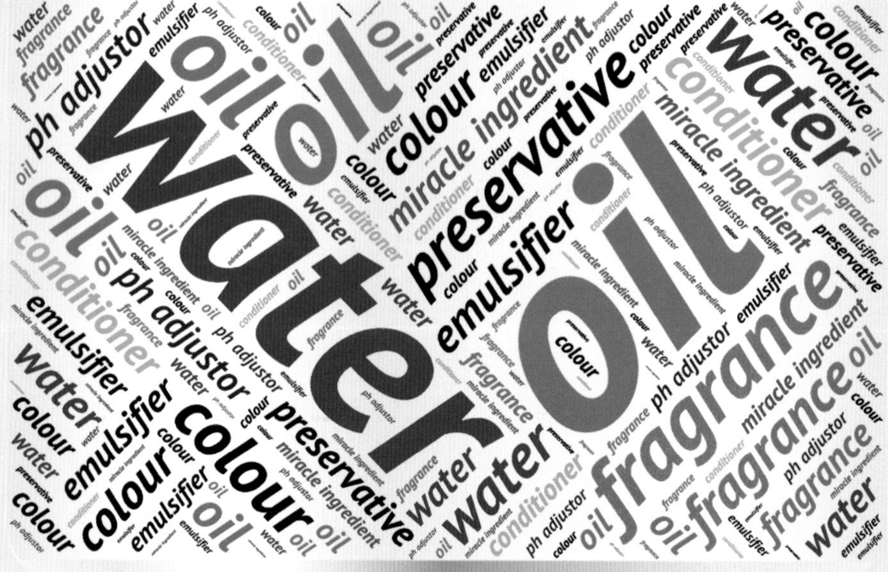
water
oil
preservative
fragrance
colour
emulsifier
conditioner
miracle ingredient
ph adjustor

Balm

Butter Oil

Natural Stabiliser

Appendix 8

How to Read an Ingredients Label

How to Read an Ingredients Label

instructions - smooth skin
Apply to body and face as required, paying particular attention to scars.
Caution: natural ingredients - may stain.
ingredients
Vitis vinifera (Grapeseed Oil)*, Hypericum perforatum (St John's Wort Oil)*, Calendula officinalis (Calendula Oil)*, Cocos Nucifera (Coconut Oil), Tocopherol (Vitamin E), Santalum album (Sandalwood), Citrus aurantium amara (Neroli), Citrus nobilis (mandarin)*, D-Limonene', Linalool', Citral, Farnesol', Geraniol'
*organic ingredients, natural constituents of essential oils
100% Natural Ingredients
Batch No. 14/11/12/1
Ebenezer House ST5 2BE
www.beautydespitecancer.co.uk
100g

36M

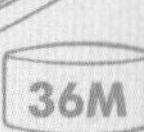

Instructions on how to use the product

Ingredients have to be written in Latin; reputable natural brands help by providing a translation; ingredients appear in concentration order, greatest first

Batch numbers allow manufacturers to trace the ingredients used in each product

This symbol illustrates the number of months within which a product should be used after it has been opened

The amount of product (weight or volume)

Manufacturer contact details

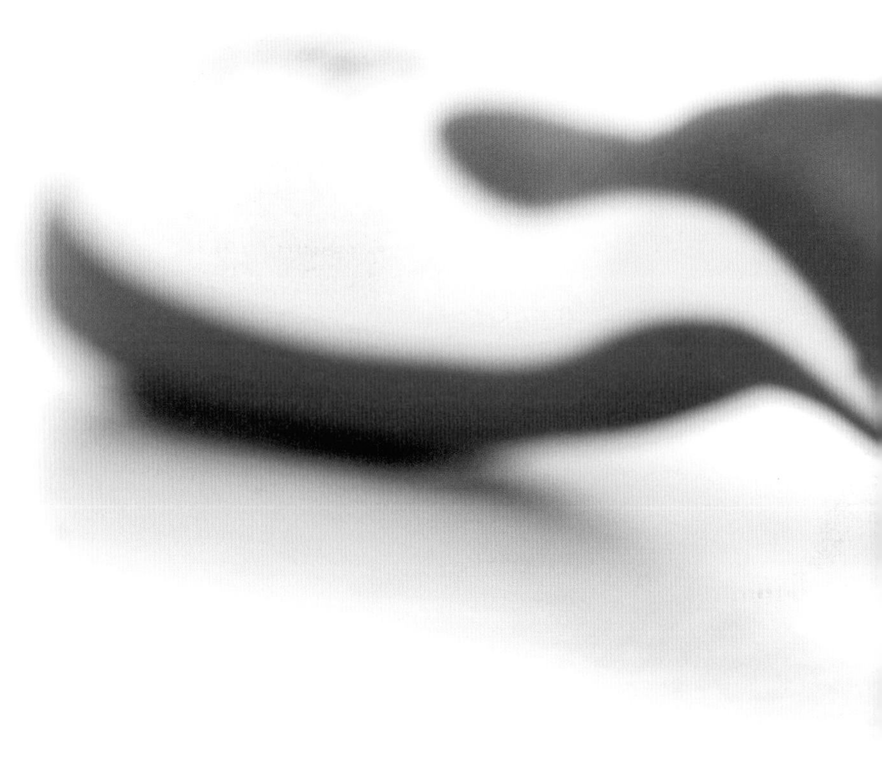

Appendix 9
Good Dental Hygiene During Treatment

Provided by Dr Chig Amin, a general dental practitioner and the founder of Epsom Dental Centre. He is the author of a special report on the early signs of mouth cancer, and has worked with the Mouth Cancer Foundation to raise awareness of mouth cancer through screenings.

- Brush your teeth every morning and evening and after every meal.
- Use a toothbrush with soft bristles.
- Replace your toothbrush every three months.
- Floss your teeth at least once a day, or as advised by your treatment team.
- Rinse your mouth five or six times a day using a bland rinse. A bland rinse is a mixture of water and sodium bicarbonate (baking soda) or a mixture of water and salt (to make a saline solution). Your treatment team will be able to advise you about the type of bland rinse suitable for you.

- Don't use a mouth rinse that contains alcohol.
- Avoid tobacco, alcohol and irritating foods, such as hot, spicy, acidic or rough foods.
- Use a moisturiser to protect your lips.
- Make sure you drink plenty of fluids throughout the day. A minimum of 1.2 litres (2 pints) is the recommended daily amount.

References

1. Frith, H., Harcourt, D. & Fussel, A. (2007). Anticipating an altered appearance: Women undergoing chemotherapy treatment for breast cancer. Eur J Oncol Nursing 11, 385–391.

2. Personal communication with Prof. Robert Thomas of Addenbrooke's Hospital, Cambridge, August 2014.

3. Massey, C.S. (2004). A multicentre study to determine the efficacy and patient acceptability of the Paxman Scalp Cooler to prevent hair loss in patients receiving chemotherapy. Eur J Oncol Nursing 8, 121–130.

4. Van den Hurk, C.J.G., Breed, W.P.M. & Nortier Short, J.W.R. (2012). Post-infusion scalp cooling time in the prevention of docetaxel-induced alopecia. Support Care Cancer 20, 3255–3260.

5. Betticher, D.C., Delmore, G., Breitenstein, U. et al. (2013). Efficacy and tolerability of two scalp cooling systems for the prevention of alopecia associated with docetaxel treatment. Support Care Cancer 21, 2565–2573.

6. Macmillan Cancer Support (2006). Worried Sick: The Emotional Impact of Cancer <available at: http://www.macmillan.org.uk/Documents/GetInvolved/Campaigns/Campaigns/Impact_of_cancer_english.pdf>.

7. Green, A. (2014). FHT Conference Presentation. An integrated approach to Complementary Therapies for Anxiety Management for Cancer Patients within the NHS – Federation of Holistic Therapists Annual Conference, Nottingham, 19th July 2014.

8. Hernandez-Reif, M., Ironson, G., Field, T., Katz, G., Diego, M., Weiss, S., Fletcher, M., Schanberg, S. & Kuhn, C. (2003). Breast cancer patients have improved immune functions following massage therapy. J Psychosom Res, 57, 45–52.

9. Hernandez-Reif, M., Field, T., Ironson, G., Beutler, J., Vera, Y., Hurley, J., Fletcher, M., Schanberg, S., Kuhn, C., & Fraser, M. (2005). Natural killer cells and lymphocytes increase in women with breast cancer following massage therapy. Int J Neurosci, 115, 495–510.

10. Listing, M., Krohn, M., Liezmann, C., Kim, I, Reisshauer, A., Peters, E., Lapp, B.F. & Rauchfuss, M. (2010). The efficacy of classical massage on stress perception and cortisol following primary treatment of breast cancer. Arch Womens Ment Health. 2010 Apr;13(2):165-173

11. Sturgeon, M., Wetta-Hall, R., Hart, T., Good, M., & Dakhil, S. (2009). Effects of therapeutic massage on the quality of life among patients with breast cancer during treatment. Journal of Complementary Medicine, 15, 373–380.

12. Rexilius, S.J., Mundt, C., Erickson Megel, M., & Agrawal, S. (2002). Therapeutic effects of massage therapy and handling touch on caregivers of patients undergoing autologous hematopoietic stem cell transplant. Oncol Nurs Forum, 29, 35–44.

13. Smith, M.C., Kemp, J., Hemphill, L., & Vojir, C.P. (2002). Outcomes of therapeutic massage for hospitalized cancer patients. J Nurs Scholarsh, 34, 257–262.

14. Soden, K., Vincent, K., Craske, S., Lucas, C., & Ashley, S. (2004). A randomized controlled trial of aromatherapy massage in a hospice setting. Palliat Med, 18, 87–92.

15. Axelsson, J., Sundelin, T., Ingre, M. et al. (2010). Beauty sleep: Experimental study on the perceived health and attractiveness of sleep deprived people. BMJ 341, c6614.

16. Dauchy, R.T., Xiang, S., Mao, L. et al. (2014). Circadian and melatonin disruption by exposure to light at night drives intrinsic resistance to tamoxifen therapy in breast cancer. Cancer Res 74(15), 4099–4110.

17. Innominato, P.F., Spiegel, D., Ulusakarya, A. et al. (2015). Subjective sleep and overall survival in chemotherapy-naïve patients with metastatic colorectal cancer. Sleep Med pii: S1389-9457(15)00055-6. doi: 1016/j.sleep.2014.10.022. [Epub ahead of print]

18. Iglesias Rosado, C., Villarino Marín, A.L., Martínez, J.A. et al. (2011). Importance of water in the hydration of the Spanish population, FESNAD 2010 document [in Spanish]. Nutr Hosp 26(1), 27–36.

19. Statista (2015). http://www.statista.com/statistics/302662/eye-make-up-usage-frequency-in-the-uk/

20. The Montreal Gazette, March 28, 1967. Italo Fava.

21. Thomas, R. (2011). Lifestyle and Cancer. The Facts: Learn how to live stronger for longer, 2nd edn. London: Health Education Publications.

22. Lalla, R.V., Bowen, J., Barasch, A. et al. (2014). MASCC/ISOO Clinical Practice Guidelines for the Management of Mucositis Secondary to Cancer Therapy <available at: http://www.mascc.org/mucositis-guidelines>.

23. Cancer Care, Inc. (2008). Caring for Your Skin During Cancer Treatment <available at: http://www.cancercare.org/publications/76caring_for_your_skin_during_cancer_treatment>.

24. Scotté, F., Tourani, J.-M., Banu, E. et al. (2005). Multicenter study of a frozen glove to prevent docetaxel-induced onycholysis and cutaneous toxicity of the hand. J Clin Oncol 23(19), 4424–4429.

25. Statista (2015). http://www.statista.com/statistics/303461/nail-varnish-care-usage-by-type-in-the-uk/.

26. Statista (2015). http://www.statista.com/statistics/276605/revenue-nail-salon-services-united-states/.

27. Gerrard, S. (2014). Adapting nail treatments during chemotherapy. Int Ther 107, 21.

28. Breast Cancer Care (2014). Breast prostheses, Bras and Clothes after Surgery <available at: http://www.nhs.uk/ipgmedia/National/Breast%20Cancer%20Care/assets/AConfidentChoiceBreastprosthesesbrasandclothesaftersurgeryBCC57pages.pdf>.

29. Alcorn, S.R., Balboni, M.J., Prigerson, H.G. et al. (2010). 'If god wanted me yesterday, I wouldn't be here today': Religious and spiritual themes in patients' experiences of advanced cancer. J Palliat Med 3(5), 581–588. [PubMed: 20408763]

30. Balboni, T.A., Vanderwerker, L.C., Block S.D. et al. (2007). Religiousness and spiritual support among advanced cancer patients and associations with end-of-life treatment preferences and quality of life. J Clin Oncol 25(5), 555–560. [PubMed: 17290065]

31. Astrow, A.B., Wexler, A., Texeira, K. et al. (2007). Is failure to meet spiritual needs associated with cancer patients' perceptions of quality of care and their satisfaction with care? J Clin Oncol 25(36), 5753–5757. [PubMed: 18089871]

32. Whitford, H.S., Olver, I.N. & Peterson, M.J. (2008). Spirituality as a core domain in the assessment of quality of life in oncology. Psycho-Oncology 17(11), 1121–1128. [PubMed: 18322902]

33. Prince-Paul, M. (2008). Relationships among communicative acts, social well-being, and spiritual well-being on the quality of life at the end of life in patients with cancer enrolled in hospice. J Palliat Med 11(1), 20–25. [PubMed: 18370887]

34. Johnson, M.E., Piderman, K.M., Sloan, J.A. et al. (2007). Measuring spiritual quality of life in patients with cancer. J Support Oncol 5(9), 437–442. [PubMed: 18019851]

35. Weaver, A.J. & Flannelly, K.J. (2004). The role of religion/spirituality for cancer patients and their caregivers. South Med J 97(12), 1210–1214. [PubMed: 15646759]

36. McCoubrie, R.C. & Davies, A.N. (2006). Is there a correlation between spirituality and anxiety and depression in patients with advanced cancer? Support Care Cancer 14(4), 379–385. [PubMed: 16283208]

37. Jenkins, R.A. & Pargament, K.I. (1995). Religion and spirituality as resources for coping with cancer. J Psychosoc Oncol 13, 51–74.

38. Thoresen, C.E. (1998). Spirituality, Health, and Science: The coming revival? The emerging role of counselling psychology in health care. New York: W.W. Norton, 409–431.

39. de Carvalho, G., Camilo, M.E. & Ravasco, P. (2011). What is the relevance of nutrition in oncology? Acta Med Port 24 Suppl 4, 1041–1050.

40. Lis, C.G., Gupta, D., Lammersfeld, C.A. et al. (2012). Role of nutritional status in predicting quality of life outcomes in cancer – A systematic review of the epidemiological literature. Nutrition J 11, 27.

41. Marín Caro, M.M, Laviano, A. & Pichard, C. (2007). Impact of nutrition on quality of life during cancer. Curr Opin Clin Nutr Metab Care 10(4), 480–487.

42. Gröber, U. (2009). Antioxidants and other micronutrients in complementary oncology. Breast Care 4, 13–20.

43. Ravasco, P., Monteiro-Grillo, I., Vidal, P.M. & Camilo, M.E. (2005). Dietary counselling improves patient outcomes: A prospective, randomized, controlled trial in colorectal cancer patients undergoing radiotherapy. J Clin Oncol 23(7), 1431–1438.

44. Ko, K., Park, Y.H., Lee, J.W. et al. (2013). Influence of nutritional deficiency on prognosis of renal cell carcinoma (RCC). BJU Int 112(6), 775–780.

45. Pan, H., Cai, S., Ji, J. et al. (2013). The impact of nutritional status, nutritional risk, and nutritional treatment on clinical outcome of 2248 hospitalized cancer patients: A multi-center, prospective cohort study in Chinese teaching hospitals. Nutr Cancer 65(1), 62–70.

46. Nicolson, G.L. & Conklin, K.A. (2008). Reversing mitochondrial dysfunction, fatigue and the adverse effects of chemotherapy of metastatic disease by molecular replacement therapy. Clin Exp Metastasis 25(2), 161–169.

47. Delia, P., Sansotta, G., Donato, V. et al. (2007). Use of probiotics for prevention of radiation-induced diarrhoea. Tumori 93(Suppl), 1–6.

48. Loh, S.Y., Ong, L., Ng, L.L. et al. (2011). Qualitative experiences of breast cancer survivors on a self-management intervention: 2-year post-intervention. Asian Pac J Cancer Prev 12(6), 1489–1495.

49. Hewitt, M.S., Greenfield, S. & Stovall, E. (Eds.) (2006). From Cancer Patient to Cancer Survivor: Lost in transition. Washington, DC: Institute of Medicine, The National Academies Press.

50. Ivers, M., Dooley, B. & Bates, U. (2009). Development, implementation and evaluation of a multidisciplinary cancer rehabilitation programme: The CANSURVIVOR Project: meeting post-treatment cancer survivors, needs. Dublin: HSE. [doi: http://hdl.handle.net/10197/2888]

51. McCabe, M.S., Bhatia, S., Oeffinger, K.C. et al. (2013). American Society of Clinical Oncology statement: Achieving high-quality cancer survivorship care. J Clin Oncol 31(5), 631–640.

52. National Cancer Survivorship Initiative <http://www.ncsi.org.uk/>.

53. Hubbard, G., Kidd, L. & Kearney, N. (2010). Disrupted lives and threats to identity: The experiences of people with colorectal cancer within the first year following diagnosis. Health 14(2), 131–146.

54. Brennan, J. (2004). Cancer in Context: A practical guide to supportive care. Oxford: Oxford University Press.

55. Rowland, J. (2006). Cancer survivorship: A new challenge in delivering quality cancer care. J Clin Oncol 24(32), 5101–5104.

56. Grassi, L. & Travado, L. (2008). The role of psychosocial oncology in cancer care. In M. Coleman, D. Alexe, T. Albrecht, & M. McKee (Eds.), Responding to the Challenge of Cancer in Europe. Slovenia: Institute of Public Health of the Republic of Slovenia.

57. Stanton, A.L. (2006). Psychosocial concerns and interventions for cancer survivors. J Clin Oncol 24(32), 5132–5137.

58. Taylor, S.E. (1983). Adjustment to threatening events: A theory of Cognitive Adaptation. Am Psychol 38, 1161–1173.

59. Stanton, A.L, Rowland, J.H., & Ganz, P.A. (2015). Life after diagnosis and treatment of cancer in adulthood: Contributions from psychosocial oncology research. Am Psychol, 70(2), 159.

60. Tomich, P.L. & Helgeson, V.S. (2004). Is finding something good in the bad always good? Benefit finding among women with breast cancer. Health Psychol 23(1), 16–23.

61. Adler, N. & Page, A. (Eds.) (2008). Cancer Care for the Whole Patient: Meeting psychosocial health needs. Washington, DC: Institute of Medicine, The National Academies Press.

62. Thoits, P.A. (2011). Mechanisms linking social ties and support to physical and mental health. J Health Soc Behav 52(2), 145–161.

63. Ganz, P.A., Desmond, K.A., Leedham, B. et al. (2002). Quality of life in long-term, disease-free survivors of breast cancer: A follow-up study. J Natl Cancer Inst 94(1), 39–49.

64. Snyder, C. (Ed.) (2000). The Handbook of Hope: Theory, measures and applications. San Diego, CA: Academic Press.

65. Snyder, C.R., Lehman, K.A., Kluck, B. & Monsson, Y. (2006). Hope for rehabilitation and vice versa. Rehabil Psychol 51(2), 89–112.

66. Chi, G.C. (2007). The role of hope in patients with cancer. Oncol Nurs Forum 34(2), 415–424.

67. Personal communication and callers to the Beauty Despite Cancer Appearance Advice Line.

Acknowledgements

This has been the hardest part of the book to write as there are so many people that I want to thank, wholeheartedly, for their generosity, kindness, influence, suggestions and help. I couldn't decide where to begin until I realised that the beginning is a good place to start.

Once upon a time, many years ago, some lovely ladies asked me for help. We worked together to make something good and that was the start. Soon, more and more people wanted to be involved, to share their good work and to help others. The writers for www.BeautyDespitecancer.co.uk (believe me, there are too many to mention) have been a hugely positive influence and have informed a lot of the content of this book – to them, and all that follow, my thanks.

I thought that I should write a book but I had no idea how to find a publisher. Don't things happen when we least expect it? As a result of a tweet sent to a fellow exhibitor at London's CAMEXPO - I have the best publisher a control freak author could ever wish for. Jon Hutchings of Lotus Publishing is relaxed and just the publisher for me. He has allowed me content and design freedom and I really hope that it turns out to be a good decision for him. It was brave of him to want to publish something on cancer beauty and well-being at a time (more than two years before publication) when there was just me and my determination to make things better.

Almost as soon as I started writing, I knew that the book needed more voices. Once again, I received help and support. The contributors to this book can all be found on my website. They have been generous with their expertise and the book is better for their involvement.

I smile as I remember thinking that writing meant job done. Oh how little I knew! How naïve I was, thinking that I could use anything other than unique images of real women living with and beyond cancer. Thanks to all of the people who helped me to realise the error of my ways via the Beauty Despite Cancer Facebook page; particular thanks to Anikka Burton of www.notanotherbunchofflowers.com. Her insistence that I had to use real models has taken this book to another level.

On to 'the shoot' – go and read Appendix 1 about the amazing professionals who gave their time and never once (at least not to my face) complained about being led by an amateur. I loved the photo shoot. I hadn't designed and managed one before and I am NEVER doing it again, but I loved it and the images make me smile every day.

When challenged to create a cover image using 'real women' I thought that I would struggle to find anyone living with or beyond cancer that would model. I was wrong! I was inundated with models and, as you can see, have a book of images, not just a cover. I haven't included their stories or even names herein. Those who want to tell their stories have done so via Beauty Despite Cancer and the press. I can, however, thank my friends Teens Unite (http://teensunitefightingcancer.org), Mummy's Star (http://www.mummysstar.org) and Sam Reynolds (http://samspaces.co.uk) for helping to spread the word about the shoot. Sam – extra thanks for driving your party bus in our direction. I have many new friends as a result of the shoot and I am honoured to have been able to work with the team who came together on that day.

The shoot was over, I had words (thanks Joy Garner for proofing and editing – how do you do that?), images and a picture in my head of what the book should look like. You cannot begin to imagine the patience and skill shown by the design team in teasing the picture from my head and making it real. Joojo Kyei-Sarpong and Martin Young, I salute you. Rest easy gentlemen, I am not writing another book … ever.

Jennifer Young

June 2015

Index